100 CHEST X-RAY PROBLEMS

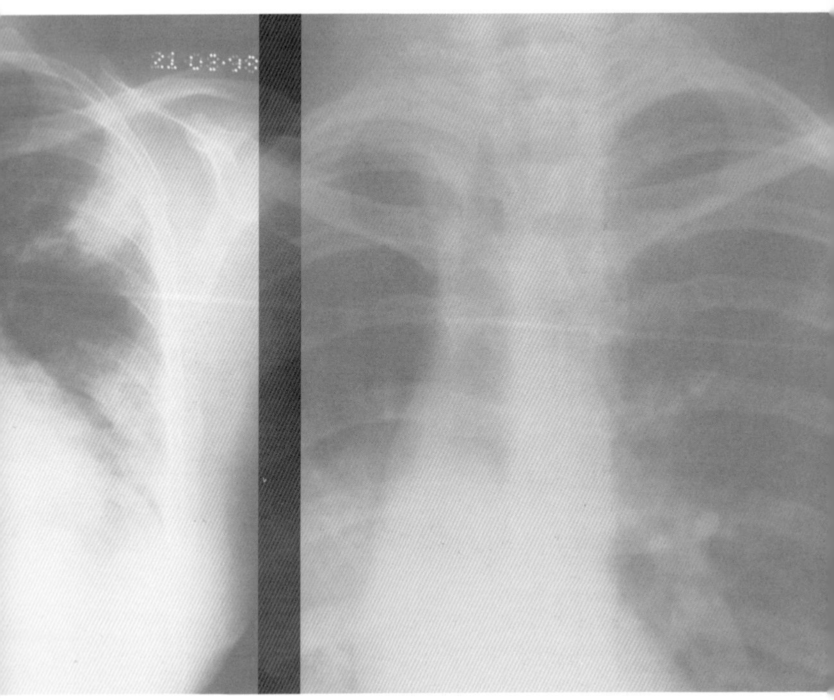

Commissioning Editor: Laurence Hunter
Development Editor: Ailsa Laing
Project Manager: Emma Riley
Designer: Stewart Larking
Illustration Manager: Gillian Murray
Illustrator: Chartwell

100 CHEST X-RAY PROBLEMS

Jonathan Corne MA PhD FRCP

Consultant Respiratory Physician,
Nottingham University Hospitals NHS Trust,
Nottingham, UK

Kate Pointon MRCP FRCR

Consultant Radiologist, Department of Radiology,
Nottingham University Hospitals NHS Trust,
Nottingham, UK

CHURCHILL LIVINGSTONE

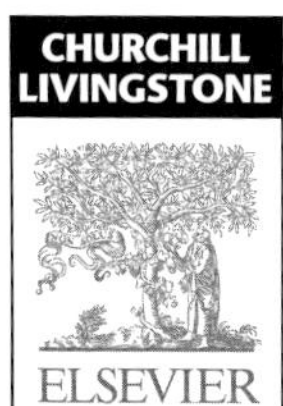

Edinburgh London New York Oxford Philadelphia St Louis Sydney Toronto 2007

CHURCHILL
LIVINGSTONE
ELSEVIER

First published 2006

ISBN 0-443-07012-1
ISBN-13 978-0-443-07012-9

International Edition ISBN 0-443-10377-1
International Edition ISBN-13 978-0-443-10377-3

British Library Cataloguing in Publication Data
A catalogue record for this book is available from the British Library

Library of Congress Cataloging in Publication Data
A catalog record for this book is available from the Library of Congress

Notice
Neither the Publisher nor the Authors assume any responsibility for any loss or injury and/or damage to persons or property arising out of or related to any use of the material contained in this book. It is the responsibility of the treating practitioner, relying on independent expertise and knowledge of the patient, to determine the best treatment and method of application for the patient.

The Publisher

The Publisher's policy is to use **paper manufactured from sustainable forests**

Printed in China

Preface

The chest X-ray is one of the most frequently requested hospital investigations. The accompanying book, 'The Chest X-Ray Made Easy', describes a simple approach to the interpretation of the chest X-ray. This new book aims to test this approach and allow you to refine your skills with a series of plain films. Some are simple, straightforward examples of X-ray abnormalities, whereas others are more complicated with multiple pathologies and less than perfect technical quality. This is deliberate, because these are the types of films you will see on the wards, and this book should therefore increase your confidence in X-ray interpretation in the real life situation.

This book contains 100 plain X-rays, mainly posteroanterior, but with some lateral projections. They are arranged in order of difficulty with the most straightforward at the beginning and the most difficult at the end. If you are able to successfully interpret the more difficult X-rays you are doing extremely well!

Good luck!

J. C.
K. P.

Nottingham
2006

Acknowledgements

With thanks to Dr. Don Rose, who provided several of the X-rays featured in this book.

CXR 1

This previously fit woman developed a dry cough following an influenza vaccination. Her general practitioner (GP) organized this film when the cough failed to clear despite antibiotic treatment. What is the abnormality on the film and what is the differential diagnosis?

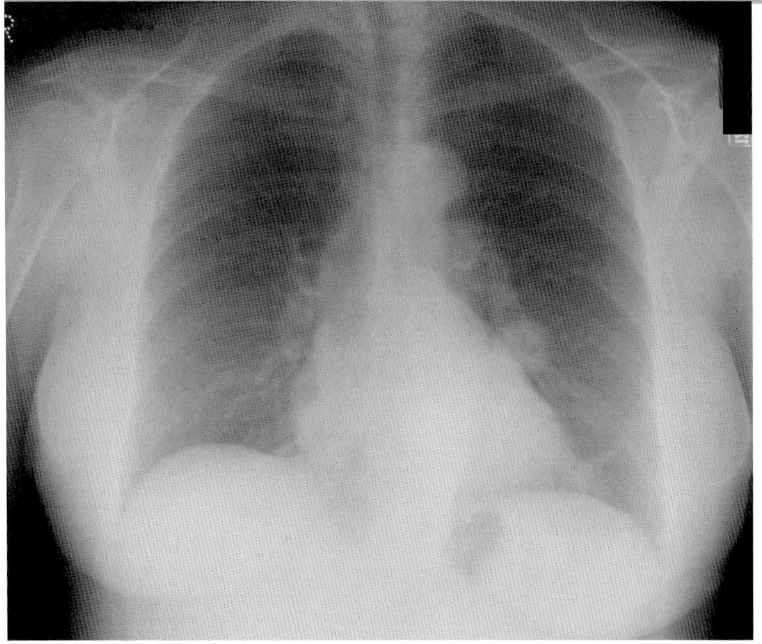

Initial impression

Area of whiteness in left lung.

Interpretation

There is an abnormal area of whiteness in the left lung field, which is adjacent to the heart border. It is a well-defined circular lesion and the whiteness is homogeneous in nature. The location of this lesion next to the heart border suggests its position is in the lingular lobe.

Solitary round lesions such as this are termed coin lesions. The differential diagnosis is very wide. The major concern would be that it is a primary lung cancer or a single secondary from another primary carcinoma. Other possibilities include a benign tumour such as a hamartoma, a rheumatoid nodule or a patch of infection. When you see a coin lesion you should look carefully for areas of calcification since this would make it more likely to be benign. Also look carefully at the nature of the whiteness. Look for an air bronchogram, which would make you think of infection, and look for an area of blackness within the white lesion, which would suggest cavitation. In this case there are no signs of cavitation and no air bronchogram.

Unfortunately this woman had a solitary adenocarcinoma metastasis. More detailed questioning revealed a history of change of bowel habit. She was found to have a primary colon cancer.

SUMMARY

Coin lesion due to secondary adenocarcinoma.

CXR 2

This is the film of a 69-year-old woman who presented to her GP with several episodes of haemoptysis. What does it show?

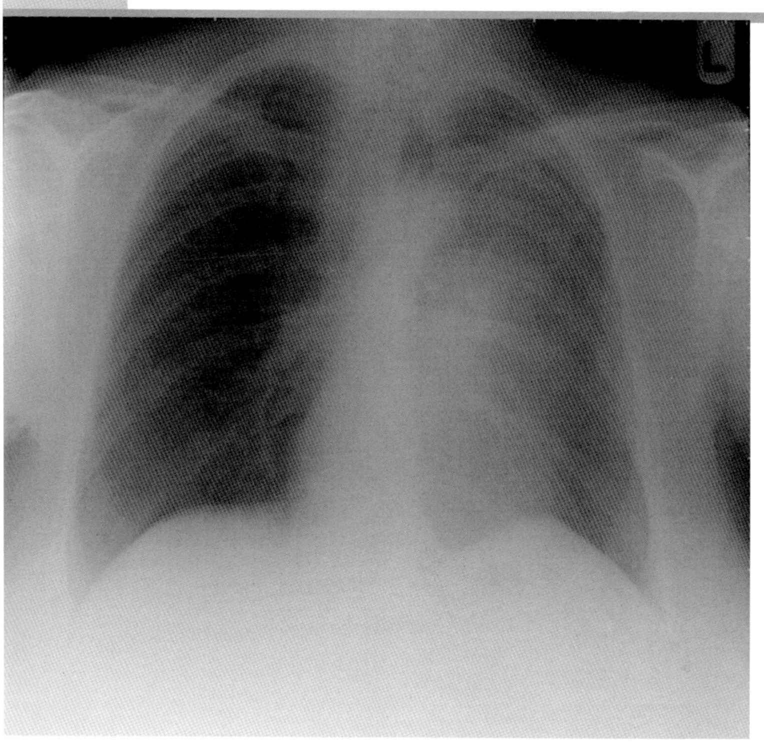

Initial impression

White left lung.

Interpretation

The left lung is white. There is no air bronchogram so this is unlikely to be consolidation. There is a loss of volume in the left lung with tracheal shift. The diaphragms are clear but the left hemidiaphragm does not have a smooth curve, and instead is peaked centrally (arrow). These features show left upper lobe collapse, which is described as a veil-like opacity over the left lung field. An obstructive malignancy in the left upper lobe bronchus is highly likely and the next investigation should be bronchoscopy and a staging computed tomography (CT) scan. In this case bronchoscopy confirmed the presence of a tumour obstructing the left upper lobe.

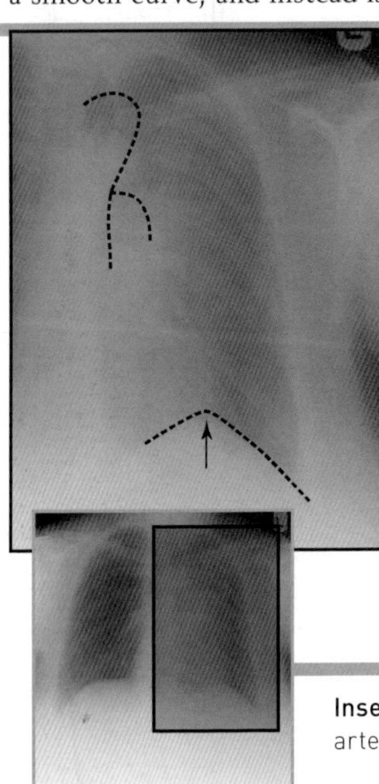

Inset: Contours of the aortic arch and pulmonary artery are lost.

SUMMARY

Left upper lobe collapse.

CXR 3

This 26-year-old post-partum woman developed breathing difficulties and needed ventilation within 24 hours of presentation. What is the likely diagnosis?

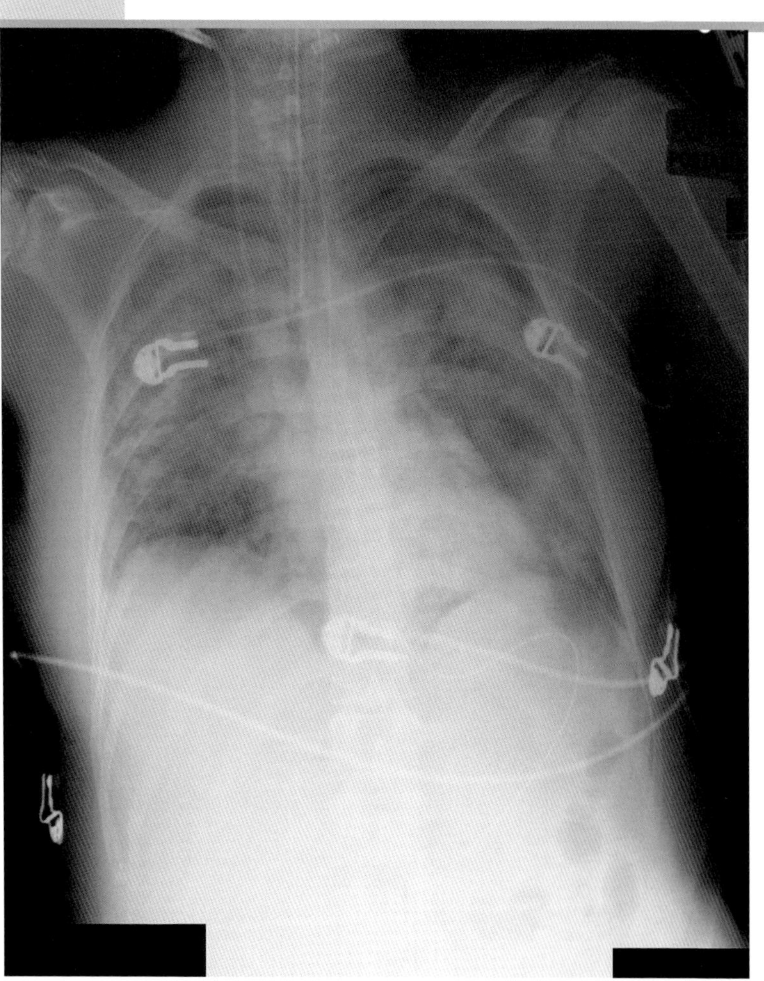

Initial impression

Increased whiteness in both lungs.

Interpretation

A brief initial inspection allows you to pick up the presence of the endotracheal tube, nasogastric tube and electrocardiogram (ECG) leads. There is a right jugular line with the tip lying below the medial end of the clavicle, and which is therefore in the correct position. This woman is obviously very unwell.

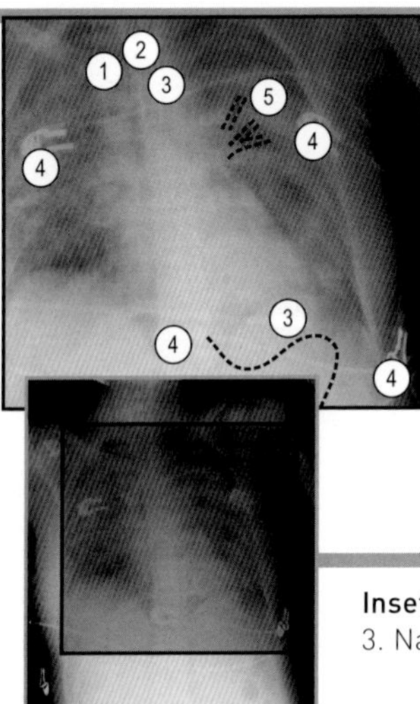

Within the lungs can be seen patchy air space change, which is quite extensive. Some blacker, linear areas within this represent the patent airways – air bronchograms. In this clinical setting the differential would include acute respiratory distress syndrome (ARDS). Pneumonia is a possibility and pulmonary haemorrhage should also be considered.

Inset: 1. Right jugular line. 2. Endotracheal tube. 3. Nasogastric tube. 4. ECG clips. 5. Bronchogram.

SUMMARY

Intubated patient, tubes and lines satisfactory, widespread airspace consolidation. Probable ARDS.

CXR 4

This 35-year-old woman presented with a 4-day history of chest pain and dyspnoea. What does the film show?

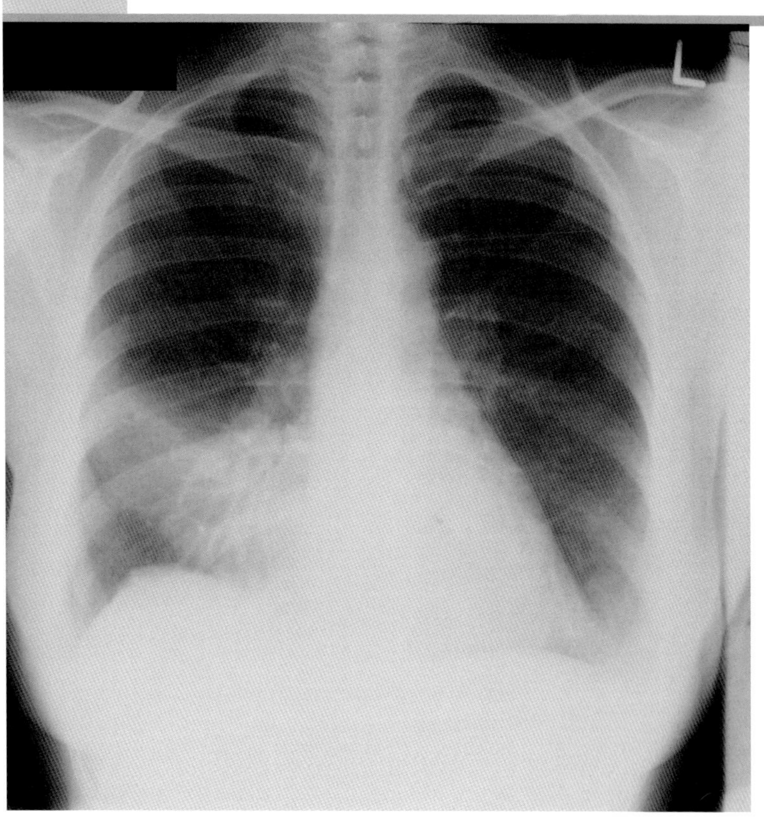

Initial impression

Abnormal whiteness in the right lung.

Interpretation

There is increased whiteness in the lower half of the right lung. This has a triangular shape with the base across the mid zone and the diagonal angled in towards the right heart border. The right hemidiaphragm remains clearly defined, so it is not the lower lobe that is involved. The right heart border, however, is not as distinct as normal, and this film shows right middle lobe pneumonia. Consolidation in the lung adjacent to a solid structure within the chest will cause that structure to lose its border. This is because the silhouette of a structure is due to the density difference between the soft tissue density heart and air-filled lungs, lost in this case because the lung air spaces are filled by consolidation.

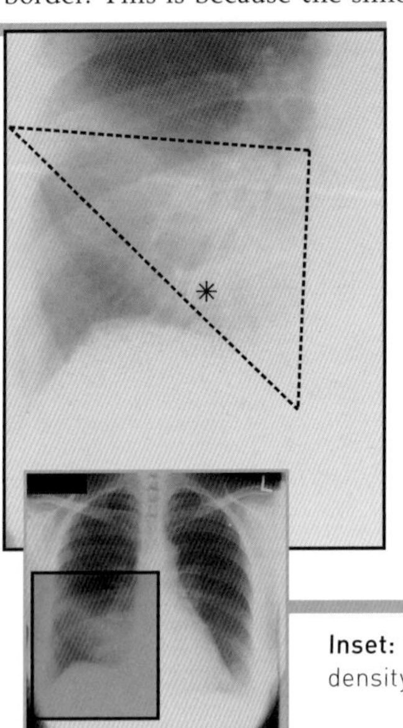

Inset: *Note how the lower border of this triangle density is straight.

SUMMARY

Right middle lobe pneumonia.

CXR 5

This is the film of a 32-year-old man who presented to the emergency department with a sudden onset of shortness of breath and right-sided pleuritic chest pain. How would you treat this patient?

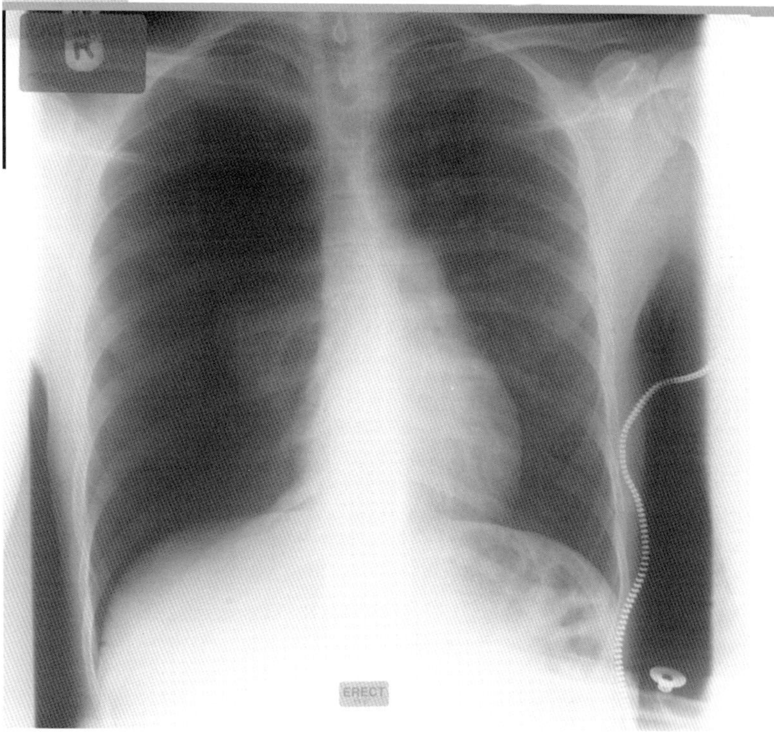

Initial impression

Black right lung field.

Interpretation

The first thing you notice when looking at this film is that the right lung field is very black. This could be due to the film being over-penetrated or a lack of lung tissue on the right due to a bulla or a pneumothorax.

The first thing you need to do is check the technical quality of the film. Look at the vertebral bodies. As you follow them down from the top of the chest they disappear behind the lower two-thirds of the heart. This means that the film is not over-penetrated. This is confirmed by looking at the left lung field, which is normal, and checking that the film is not rotated, which it is not. Therefore the blackness is not due to a technical artefact.

In a young man the most likely diagnosis of a black lung is a pneumothorax. This is confirmed in this film by the presence of the squashed lung whose outer convex boundary can be clearly seen.

In older patients a pneumothorax can be confused with an emphysematous bulla. These can be distinguished by looking at the lung edge, which in a pneumothorax is convex (as it is here), and with a bulla often concave. The nature of the blackness can also be helpful. As in this case, in a pneumothorax there are usually no visible lung markings in the area of blackness whereas with a bulla, curved fine strands can often be seen running across it.

The size of a pneumothorax is determined by measuring the distance between the lung edge and the chest wall. The pneumothorax shown here is over 2 cm and so the recommended treatment would be aspiration, or insertion of a chest drain, should aspiration be unsuccessful.

You will have also noticed the white chain-like structure adjacent to the left chest wall. This is the zip of the patient's jacket – the patient was obviously too unwell to be undressed fully before the film was taken.

SUMMARY

Right pneumothorax. Treatment by aspiration followed, if necessary, by intercostal tube drainage.

CRX 6

This 45-year-old woman presented with a chronic cough and weight loss. What diagnosis is suggested by this film?

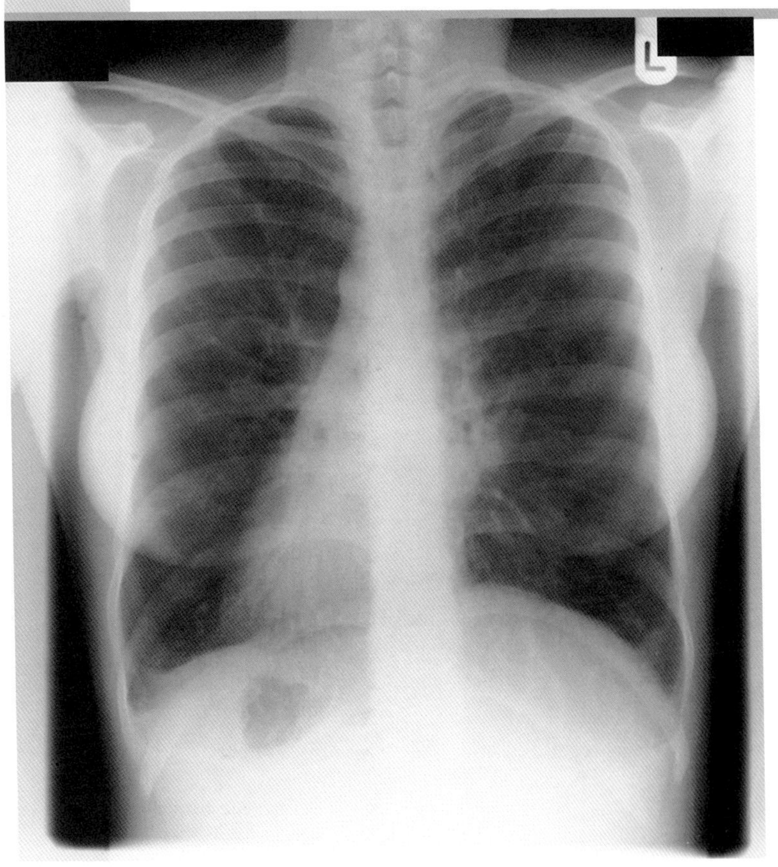

Initial impression

Abnormal mediastinum.

Interpretation

The cardiac apex is to the right of the midline and the aortic arch is also to the right. Look for the gastric bubble – this is also on the right. The patient may have situs inversus or the film may be mislabelled. You will need to examine the patient to see which is the case.

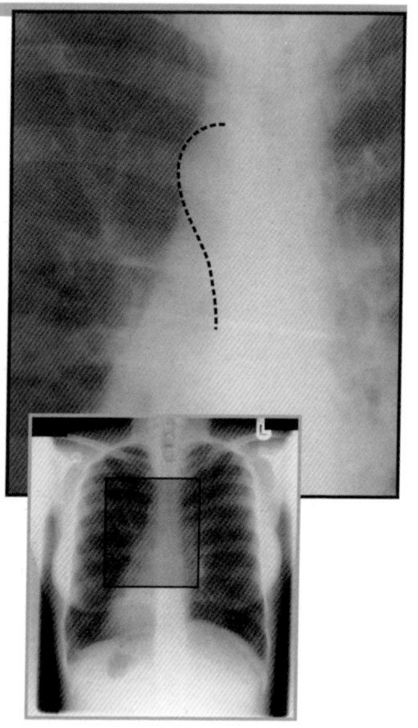

Remember not to stop examining the film the moment you discover the obvious abnormality. In this case further inspection shows the lungs to be abnormal. The lungs are large in volume and there are subtle streaky shadows in the lung fields. These streaky shadows are thickened bronchial walls and are a sign of bronchiectasis. If you look closely you will see that pairs of these lines run parallel with each other giving the appearance of a tramline. This is the appearance of diseased bronchi seen side on. An end on airway can be seen at the left base, producing a ring shadow. The patient has situs inversus and bronchiectasis – the diagnosis is Kartagener's syndrome.

SUMMARY

Kartagener's syndrome.

CXR 7

This is a lateral film of a 42-year-old man who gave a 2-week history of a cough productive of green sputum, loss of appetite and malaise. The posteroanterior (PA) film showed left mid-zone consolidation. What does the lateral tell us about the location of the pathology?

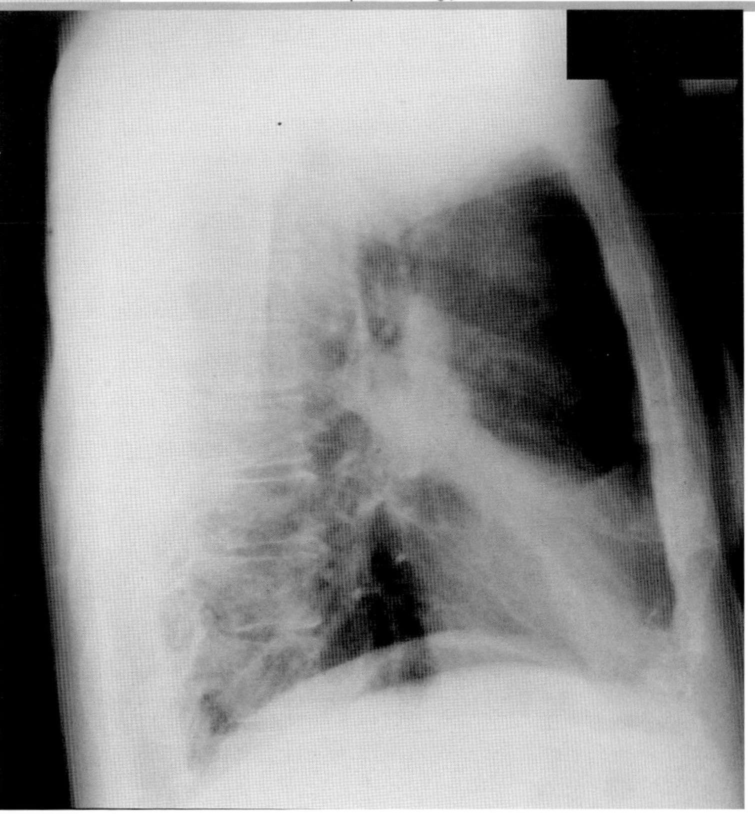

Initial impression

Area of increased whiteness.

Interpretation

This lateral film confirms that there is an area of increased whiteness in the lung, which we know from the PA film is in the left lung. The lateral can help localize the pathology to one or more lobes. In this case the increased shadowing overlies the heart, extending from the centre of the film, anteriorly and downwards, to the cardiophrenic angle. The anterior location close to the heart indicates that the whiteness lies within the lingular lobe. This patient had a lingular pneumonia.

Many clinicians are unfamiliar with looking at the lateral film. Here are a few simple rules:

1. Check the lung appearances in front of, and above the heart to the area behind. They should all be similar.
2. The area lying behind the sternum is known as the retrosternal space. This should be the darkest area of the film. Any whiteness in this region is abnormal and would suggest pathology either within the anterior portions of the upper lobes or the superior mediastinum.
3. Check the positions of the horizontal and oblique fissures if they are visible on the film.
4. Check the density of the hila; overlying masses may make them appear whiter than usual.
5. Look at the diaphragms; a small pleural effusion may be easier to identify on a lateral film.
6. Survey the thoracic spine. At the top of the film it appears very white and unclear since it is covered by the soft tissue of the shoulder girdle. As you follow the thoracic spine downwards it should gradually get easier to visualize. If this transition is lost it may indicate pathology within the lower lobes, or perhaps a pleural effusion. The vertebral bodies can also be examined and vertebral body collapse or abnormal bony density checked for.

SUMMARY

Lingular consolidation.

CXR 8

A 61-year-old woman presented to her GP with a short history of cough and increasing shortness of breath. On direct questioning she admitted to night sweats. Following auscultation of her chest, the GP ordered this film. What does it show?

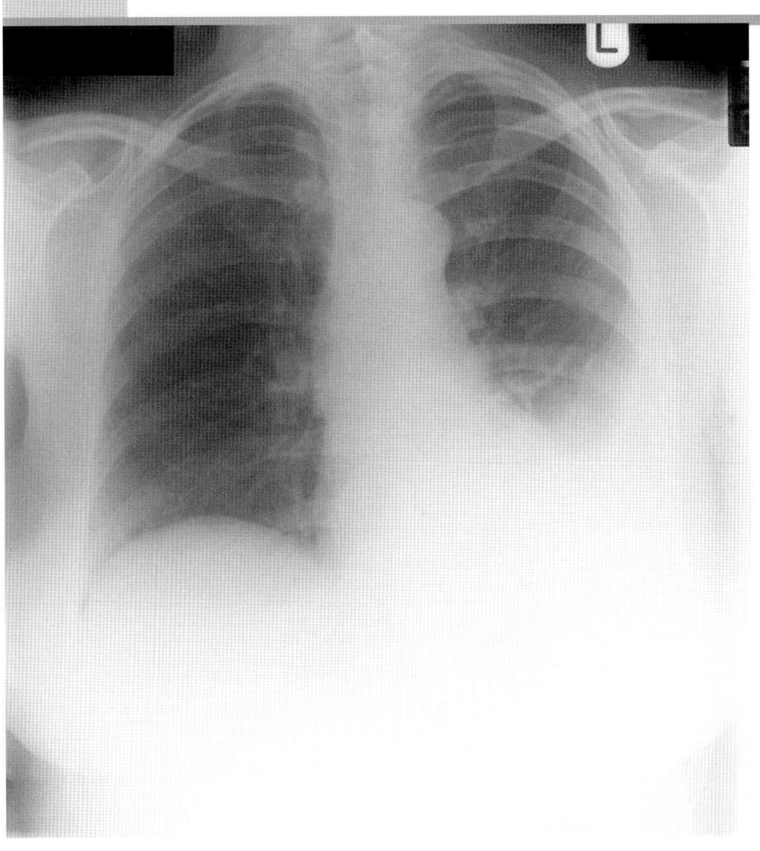

Initial impression

Area of whiteness in left lung.

Interpretation

There is a white area in the lower zone of the left lung. This is homogeneous in nature with no air bronchogram, so it is unlikely to be due to consolidation. The upper border is curved upwards like an exaggerated meniscus. This is known by radiologists as a lamellar sign. The nature of the whiteness, and the exaggerated meniscus, make a pleural effusion the most likely cause.

Always remember to look at the rest of the film for clues as to the cause of the effusion. In particular, check the position of the mediastinum since, if this has shifted towards the effusion, there may be underlying lung collapse hidden by the fluid. In this case, the rest of the film was normal.

This woman had a pleural effusion following pneumonia.

SUMMARY

Left pleural effusion.

CXR 9

This is a follow-up film of a 72-year-old ex-smoker. What is the explanation of this film appearance?

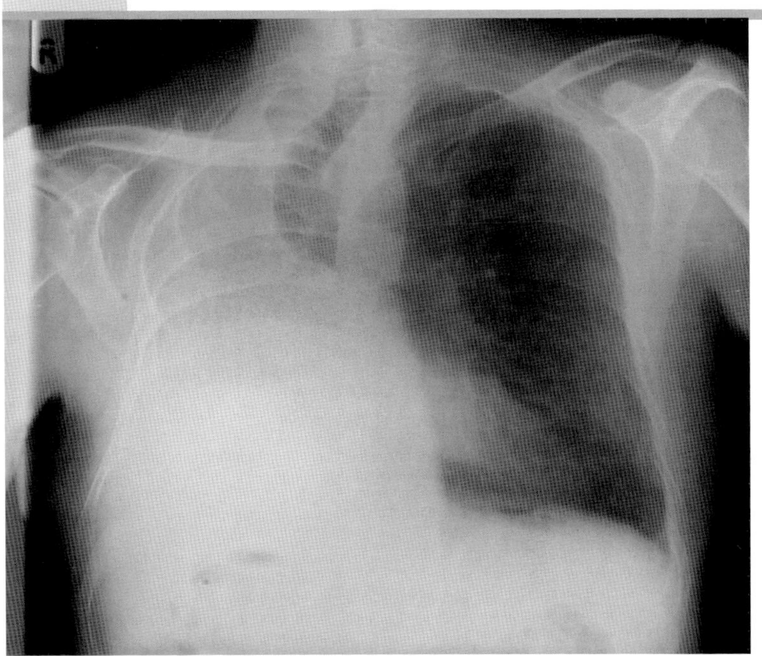

Initial impression

White right lung.

Interpretation

The right lung field is completely white and the whiteness is homogeneous in nature. If you see a 'white lung' then the possible causes are fluid as in a pleural effusion, consolidation or collapse of part or all of the lung. In this film the whiteness is homogeneous and does not demonstrate any evidence of an air bronchogram – it is therefore unlikely to be due to consolidation. If you look closely you will see that the mediastinum is shifted to the right with a prominent curve to the right of the trachea. This suggests a considerable loss of volume of the right lung. Look also at the heart. In this film the heart is not clearly visible in the left hemithorax. This is because it has been pulled to the right as the whole mediastinum has been pulled across, again suggesting considerable loss of volume on the right. The whiteness has therefore been caused by something that is reducing the volume of the lung: either collapse of the lung or a pneumonectomy. You can identify further clues from looking at other structures. If you look for bronchial markings you can see a very clear left main bronchus but no part of the right bronchial tree is visible. If you look at the bony structures you can just make out the ribs on the right side except for the 5th rib, which has been surgically resected. This patient had a right pneumonectomy for a squamous cell bronchial carcinoma involving the right main bronchus.

SUMMARY

Right pneumonectomy.

CXR 10

This 65-year-old man has had this film taken and wants to know what the implications of these changes are. What will you tell him?

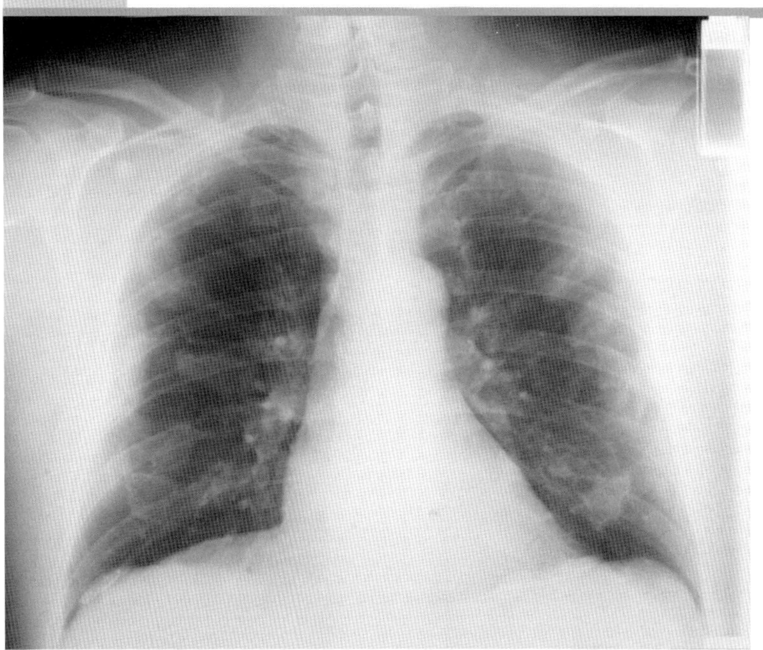

Initial impression

Abnormal white areas both lungs.

Interpretation

There are well-defined irregular densities in both hemithoraces. These appear calcified and follow the long axis of the ribs at many levels. They are asbestos related pleural plaques. They typically run along the line of the anterior portion of the ribs and the calcification is said to give them a map-like appearance. Comparison with previous films can be useful, since pleural plaques should be stable over time.

Exposure to airborne fibres of asbestos may produce problems in the lung or the pleura. Pleural plaques are the commonest radiographic presentation and are usually asymptomatic. More extensive changes, known as diffuse pleural thickening can occur and do affect breathing. Further problems include simple pleural effusions, and mesothelioma. Asbestos lung changes include asbestosis, and a recognized increase in incidence of lung cancer.

In this case, you can tell the patient that these plaques are benign, and unlikely to cause him serious problems. Asbestos exposure will have been a result of occupational exposure. In the UK, compensation may be sought through the civil courts.

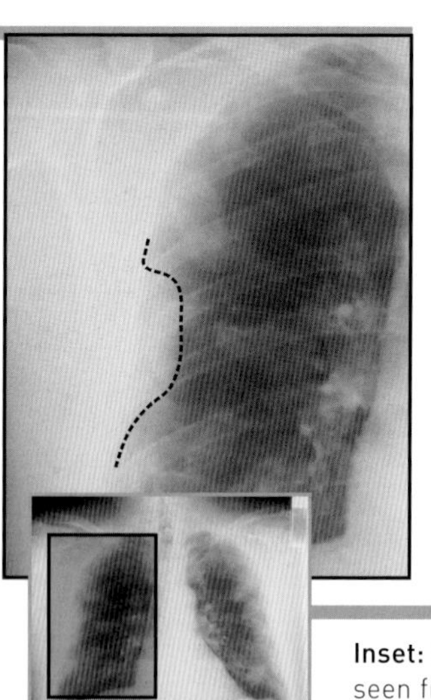

Inset: Pleural plaque against the lateral chest wall seen from the side, jutting into the lung.

SUMMARY

Extensive bilateral pleural plaques.

CXR 11

This 53-year-old woman has attended a chest clinic via her GP and is very anxious because she has recently developed a cough. The lungs on this film are clear, so why has this woman been so anxious?

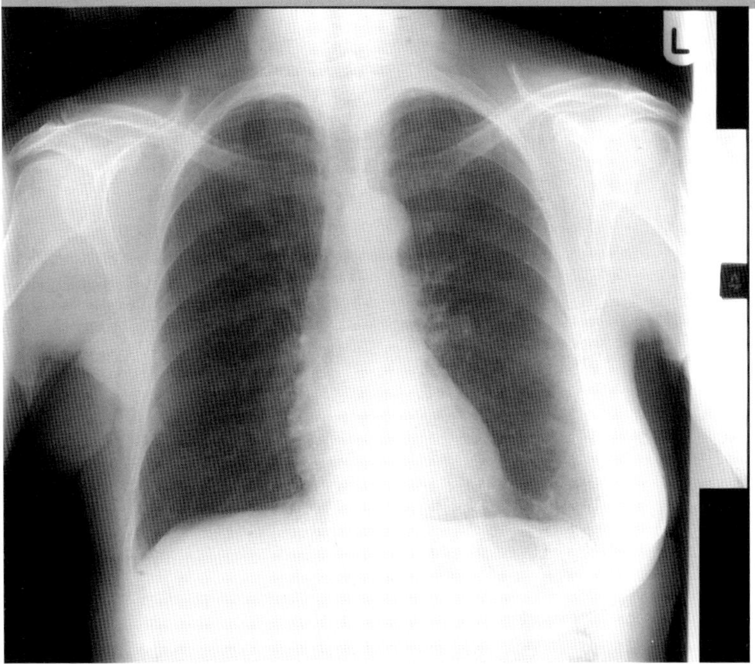

Initial impression

Normal chest film.

Interpretation

The review areas for any film must include the bones and the soft tissues. Can you identify that the lung on the right looks blacker than the lung on the left? This is because there is less overlying soft tissue as a result of a right mastectomy for breast cancer. Look at the soft tissues running up to the right axilla – you should be able to see that they are distorted and do not form a smooth curve as on the opposite side.

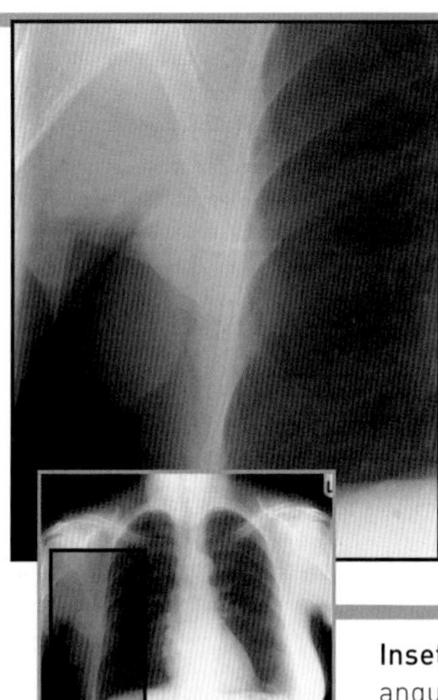

Inset: Asymmetry of the breast tissue and distorted angular folds within the axilla.

SUMMARY

Previous mastectomy. This woman has had breast cancer and was worried that her breathlessness might be due to recurrent disease, which can commonly involve the lungs, often producing a pleural effusion or lymphangitis.

CXR 12

This patient with known chronic renal failure developed a troublesome cough with increasing breathlessness. What is the cause of these symptoms?

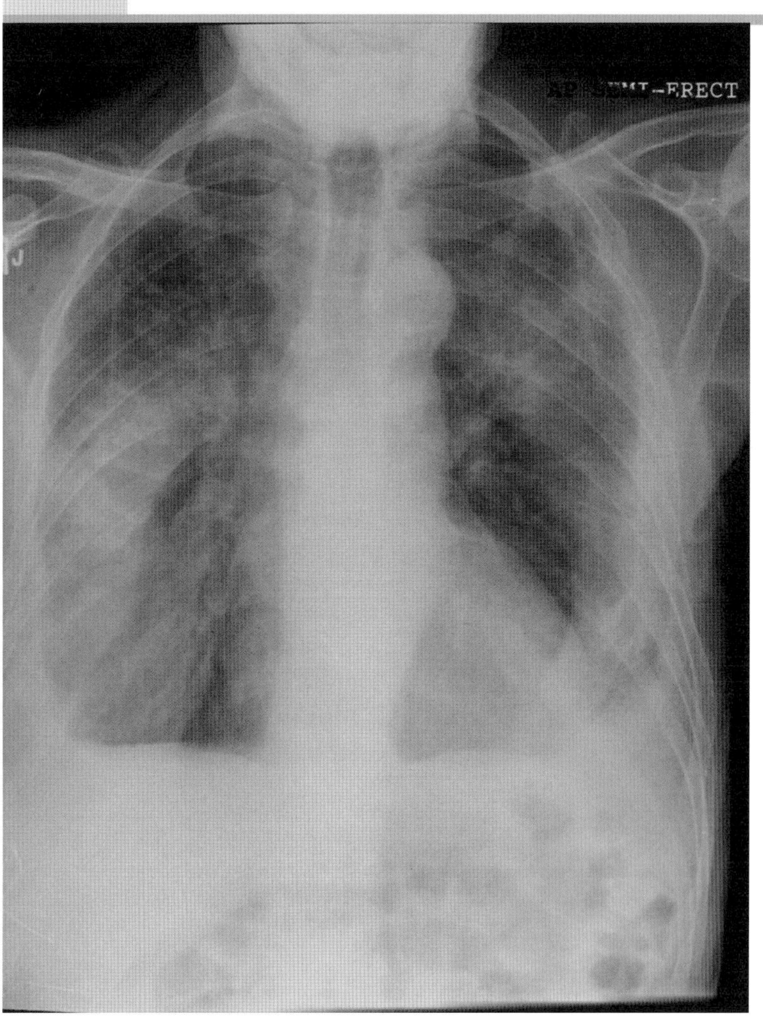

Initial interpretation

Bilateral white lung fields.

Interpretation

Initial inspection of this film shows multiple areas of white shadows. You need to examine each of these areas separately.

At the base of both hemithoraces there is a homogeneous white shadowing that is flat centrally but curves upwards at the edges like a meniscus. The normal diaphragmatic shadow is obscured. The homogeneous nature of this shadowing and the presence of a meniscus strongly suggest that this is a pleural effusion.

The second white shadow can be seen in both hemithoraces and is more complex in nature. The upper part of this shadowing is patchy in nature, which implies that the alveoli are affected, therefore suggesting that it is intrapulmonary. The lower part of the whiteness is more homogeneous and has very well-defined medial margins. The inner margin on the right is s-shaped, and on the left it is a reversed c-shape. This is the appearance caused by fluid tracking into the oblique fissures. This area of whiteness is due to bilateral pleural effusions.

The presence of bilateral pleural effusions and alveolar shadowing is very suggestive of pulmonary oedema. Therefore you should look carefully at the heart shadow since pulmonary oedema is commonly secondary to heart disease – and you may expect to see an enlarged heart. In this case the heart shadow is not enlarged and has a normal shape. The pulmonary oedema in this patient was due to fluid overload and was not cardiogenic in nature.

This is a complicated film. It demonstrates the importance of looking at the margins of the shadowing in an attempt to localize pathology to either lungs or pleura.

SUMMARY

Pulmonary oedema, secondary to fluid overload.

CXR 13

This 68-year-old woman was admitted following a collapse in the high street and required immediate intubation and ventilation. This film was taken a half hour later, just prior to her transfer to the intensive care unit. What action is required?

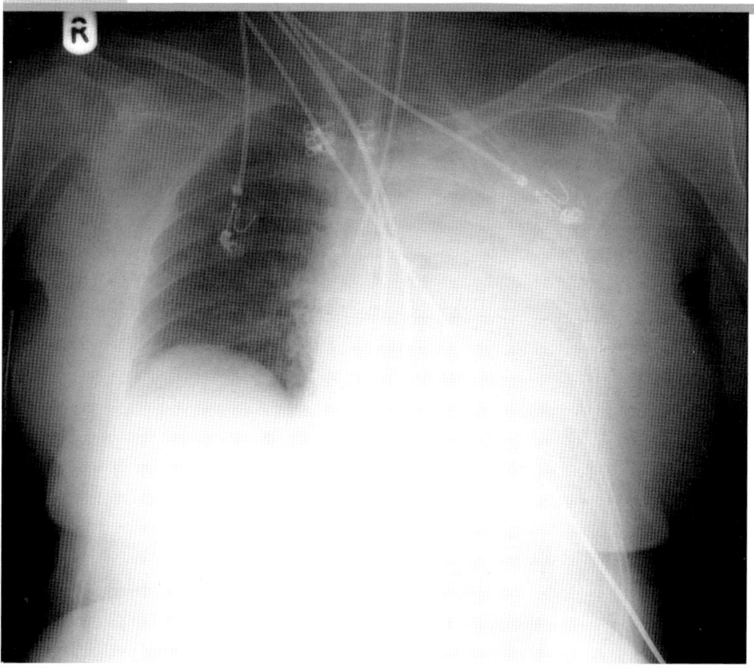

Initial impression

White left lung.

Interpretation

There are ECG leads overlying the chest and the metal hooks on the patient's bra strap are visible on the film. There is an endotracheal tube in situ. The left lung is completely white. This shadowing is homogeneous in nature. The film is rotated, but even allowing for this you can see that the endotracheal tube, which marks the position of the trachea, is shifted to the left suggesting collapse of the left lung. Follow the line of the endotracheal tube and you will see that it then deviates towards the right side of the thorax. The tube has been pushed too far and has passed into the right main bronchus. The left lung is no longer being aerated and as a result has collapsed. The endotracheal tube needs to be re-positioned so that it lies above the carina.

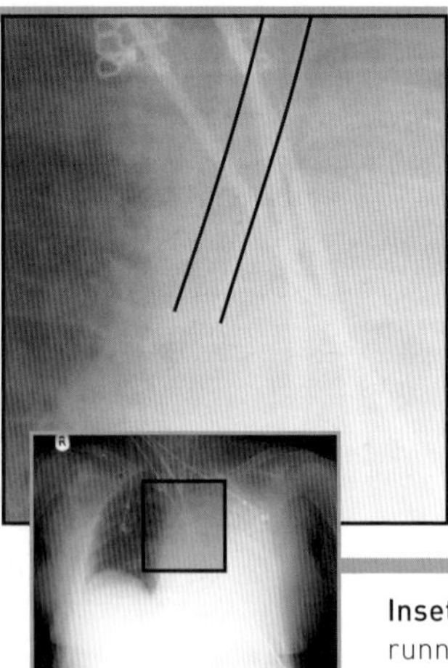

Inset: The dense white stripe is the opaque marker running down the endotracheal tube.

SUMMARY

Collapse of the left lung due to an incorrectly sited endotracheal tube. This needs to be withdrawn by around 5 cm.

CXR 14

This 62-year-old man was admitted as an emergency. His son had returned from Australia to find him unable to look after himself, not eating or drinking and obviously having lost a lot of weight. What does his film show?

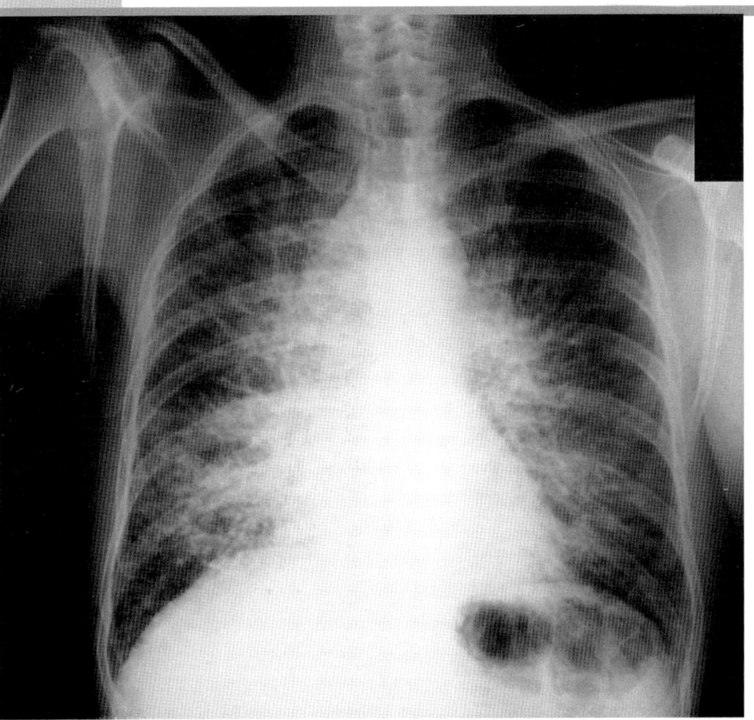

Initial impression

Bilateral white lungs.

Interpretation

There is abnormal whiteness in both lung fields. This is not homogeneous shadowing and there are no air bronchograms. You must therefore think about causes of interstitial lung disease such as pulmonary fibrosis, pulmonary oedema and lymphangitis carcinomatosis. The distribution of this shadowing gives important clues. It affects the upper, middle and lower lung zones and is central in its distribution. This would be unusual for fibrotic lung disease, which usually involves the lung periphery and bases, and would be very atypical of pulmonary oedema. Furthermore the heart size is normal which goes against pulmonary oedema. This is a common distribution for lymphangitis carcinomatosis. Causes would be primary adenocarcinoma of the pancreas, gastrointestinal tract, prostate and lung.

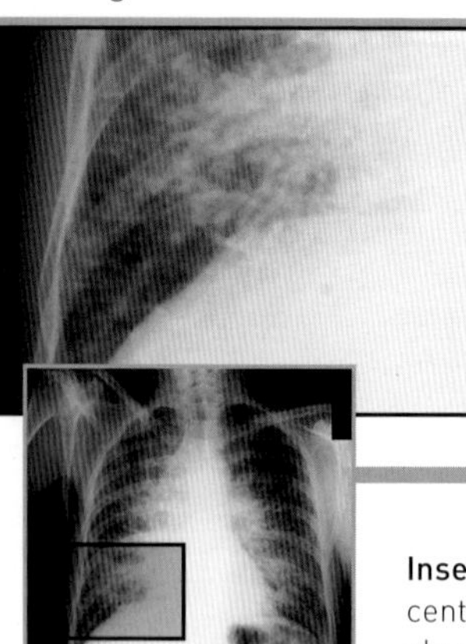

Inset: Coarse linear shadowing which is mainly central, but some shadowing extends to the lateral chest wall.

SUMMARY

Lymphangitis carcinomatosis, which on further investigation was found to be due to an underlying adenocarcinoma of the pancreas.

CXR 15

This tall, 25-year-old man was admitted to hospital after he suddenly became short of breath. What was the initial diagnosis and what treatment was instituted?

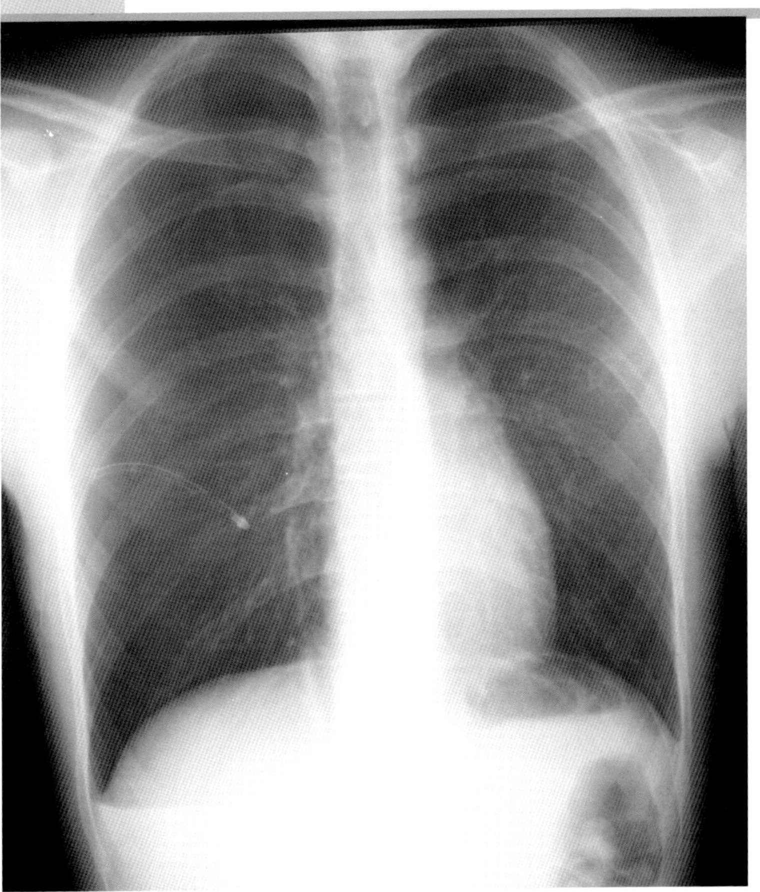

Initial impression

Black lung.

Interpretation

Looking at this film you can immediately tell that this patient is tall and slim. The right lung looks black and on closer inspection you can see the lung edge, about a quarter of the way in from the chest wall. At the bottom of the right lung you can see a white dense area with a horizontal upper border. This patient has a hydropneumothorax. The very straight upper edge to the whiteness is typical of an air/fluid interface and the visible lung edge is typical of a pneumothorax. The small tube, visible half way up the chest, is a chest drain. The air/fluid level beneath the left diaphragm is due to stomach contents in the fundus.

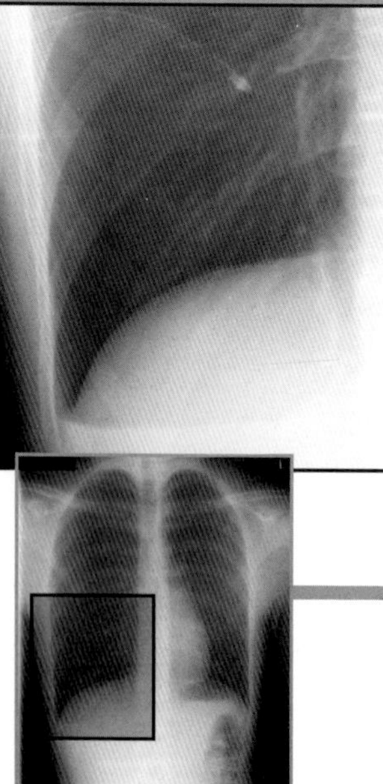

SUMMARY

Pneumothorax, treated by chest drain insertion.

CXR 16

This 64-year-old man had a 4-week history of haemoptysis. He also reported weight loss and feeling generally unwell. This film was ordered when he attended the hospital chest clinic. What does it show?

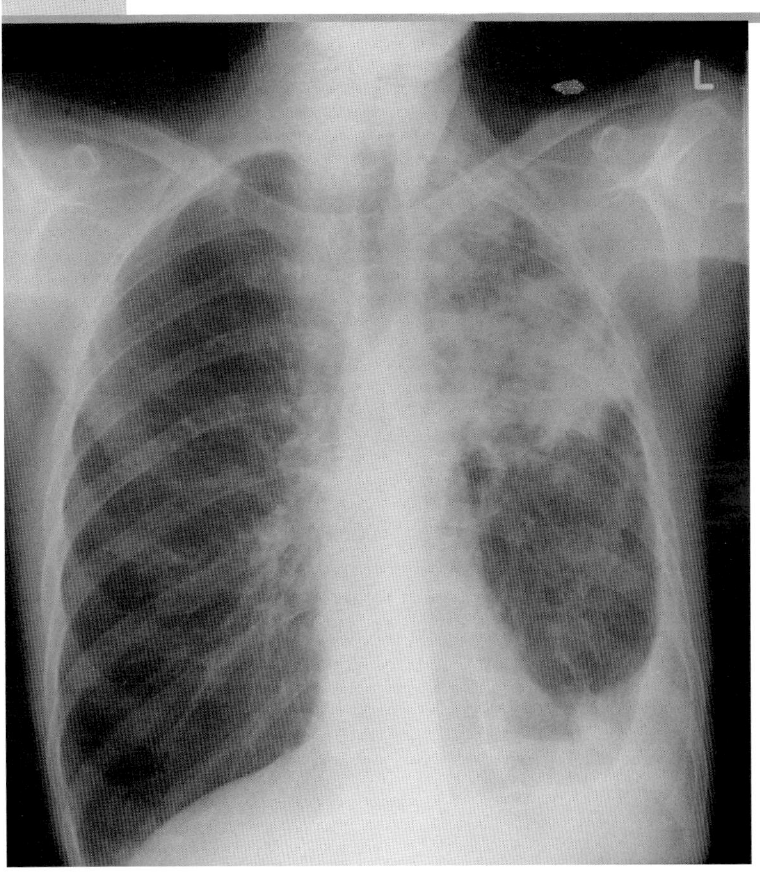

Initial impression

Areas of white lung.

Interpretation

There are two areas of whiteness in the left lung field. One is in the apex and the other in the lower zone. The lower area is homogeneous white, has an obvious meniscus and completely obscures the diaphragm – this is a pleural effusion. The area of whiteness in the upper zone is more patchy in nature. Look carefully at this area of whiteness. You can see the bronchi as black lines against the area of whiteness. This is an air bronchogram, which suggests consolidation. At the top of the lung, peripherally you can also see a small black area, which is a small cavity. This combination of apical consolidation and cavitation is very suggestive of pulmonary tuberculosis. The pleural effusion is likely also to be due to tuberculosis.

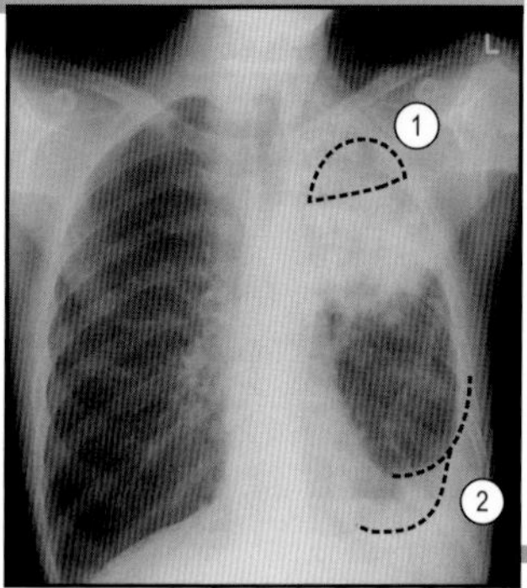

Above: 1. Area of cavitation. 2. Fluid around the base of the lung and tracking in the fissure.

SUMMARY

Pulmonary tuberculosis.

CXR 17

This 75-year-old retired nurse had this film taken as part of a private medical assessment. Is the film normal?

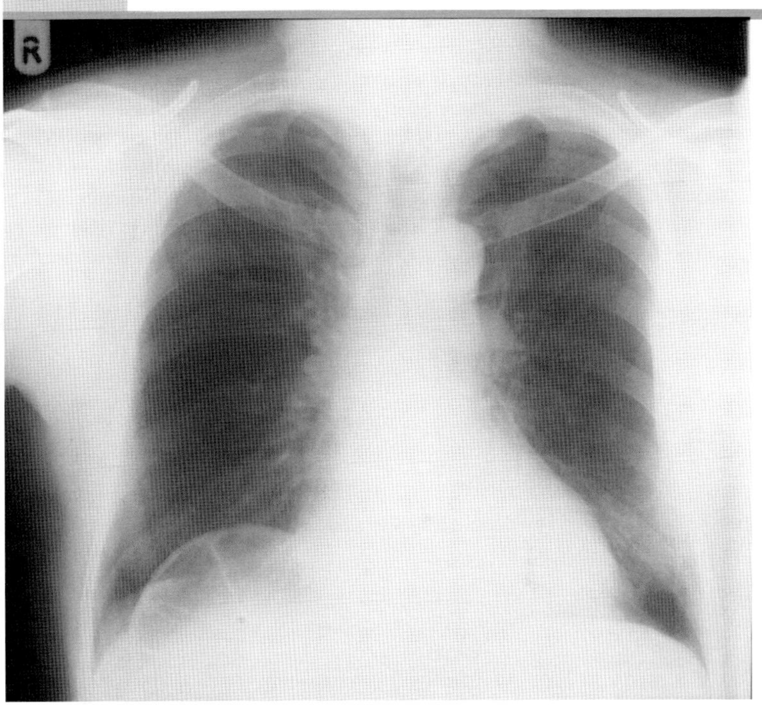

Initial impression

Abnormality under the diaphragm.

Interpretation

The lung fields, heart and mediastinum are normal, as are the soft tissues. However, further inspection suggests an unusual area under the right diaphragm. There is an area of blackness between the lower edge of the diaphragm and the liver. This could be free air under the diaphragm or air within the gut. Differentiating between the two is obviously crucial. Look carefully at the area of blackness; with free air there should not be lines crossing the blacker area. In this film you can see faint lines running almost perpendicularly from the lower edge of the diaphragm to the upper edge of the liver. This indicates that the air is within the colon and the lines represent folds (haustrae). This appearance is known as Chilaiditi's syndrome.

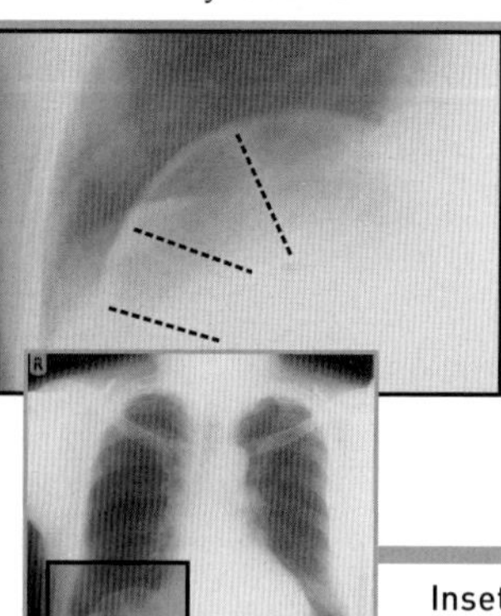

Inset: Haustrae indicating this is due to colon beneath the diaphragm.

SUMMARY

Chilaiditi's syndrome – a normal variant. This study is normal.

CXR 18

This 43-year-old man reported to his occupational health department with a persistent cough, wheeze and shortness of breath. The only history of note was of an accident at his workplace, when he fell from a loading bay the previous year. Comment on this film.

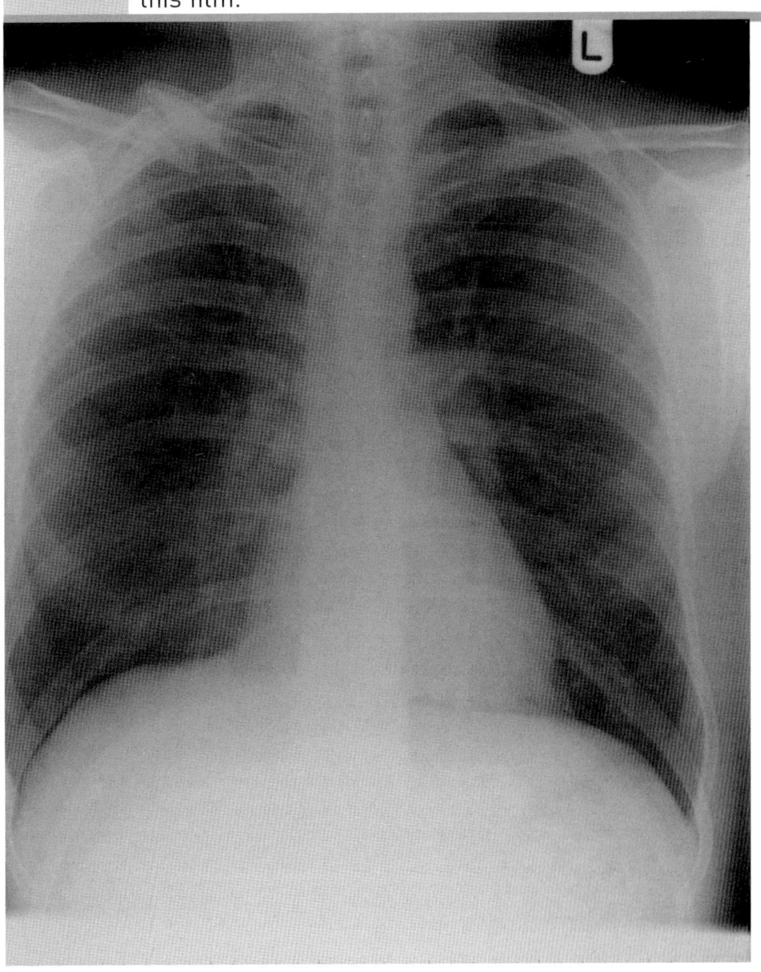

Initial impression

Fracture of the right clavicle.

Interpretation

Always remember to look at the bones and soft tissues. This man has normal lung fields and a normal heart (his symptoms were due to asthma); however, the examination of the film is not complete until you have surveyed the bones and soft tissue. The right clavicle is clearly abnormal. There is a fracture through the mid diaphysis with overlap of the bony fragments and upward displacement of the medial portion of the clavicle.

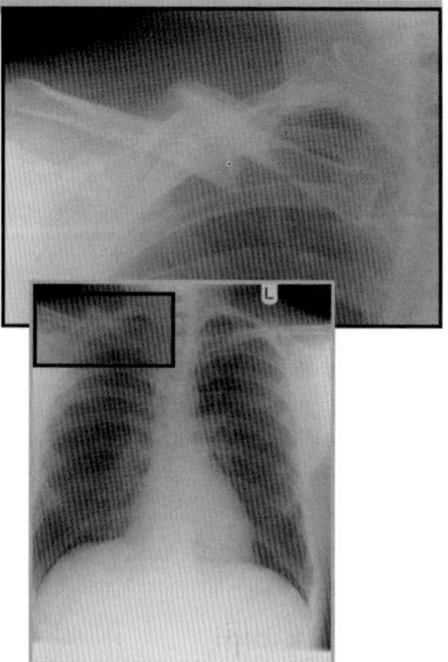

SUMMARY

Healed fracture of the right clavicle, with shortening. No cause for respiratory symptoms seen.

CXR 19

This 40-year-old man presented with an acute 2-day history of significant haemoptysis and increasing breathlessness. He was admitted to accident and emergency where this film was taken. What does the supine film show?

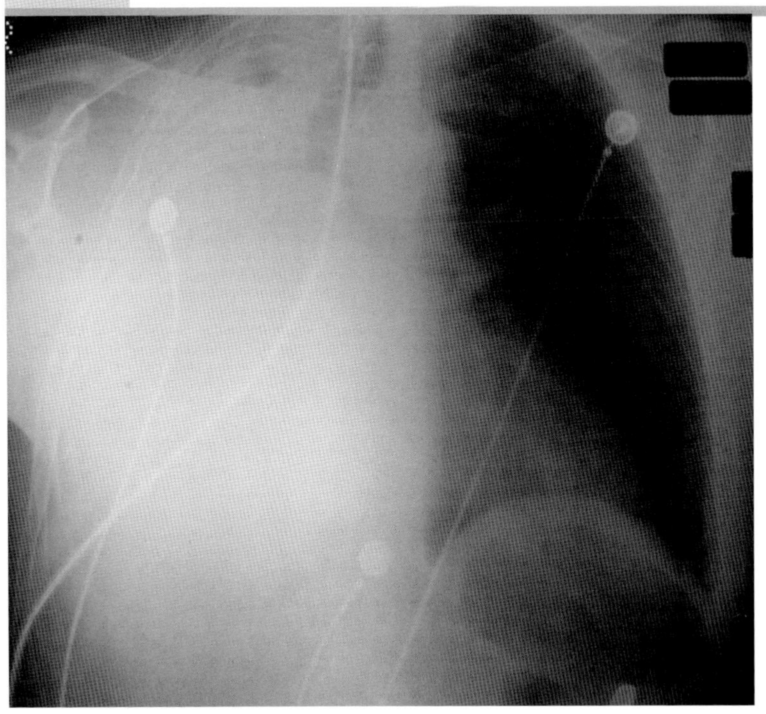

Initial impression

White lung.

Interpretation

The patient is being monitored and ECG leads are visible. The right lung is completely white. The trachea is shifted towards the right, confirming loss of volume on the right side. The trachea is easy to identify and, following it down, you can easily make out the left main bronchus. The right main bronchus cannot be seen on this film and careful examination shows a white tongue-like shadow at what should be the mouth of the right main bronchus. This implies the presence of something solid obstructing the right main bronchus, which in this case is a clot of blood. The differential diagnosis would include tumour or an inhaled foreign body.

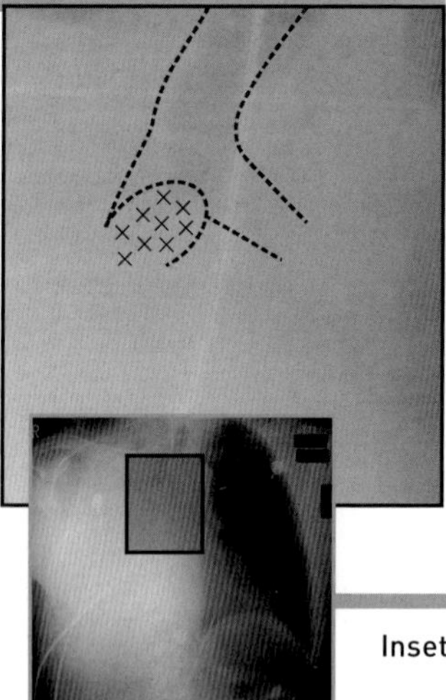

Inset: Clot in the proximal right main bronchus.

SUMMARY

Right lung collapse secondary to blockage of the right main bronchus.

CXR 20

This 20-year-old woman with acute myeloid leukaemia developed rapidly increasing shortness of breath following chemotherapy. She required transfer to intensive care where she was intubated and ventilated. What is the cause of her breathlessness?

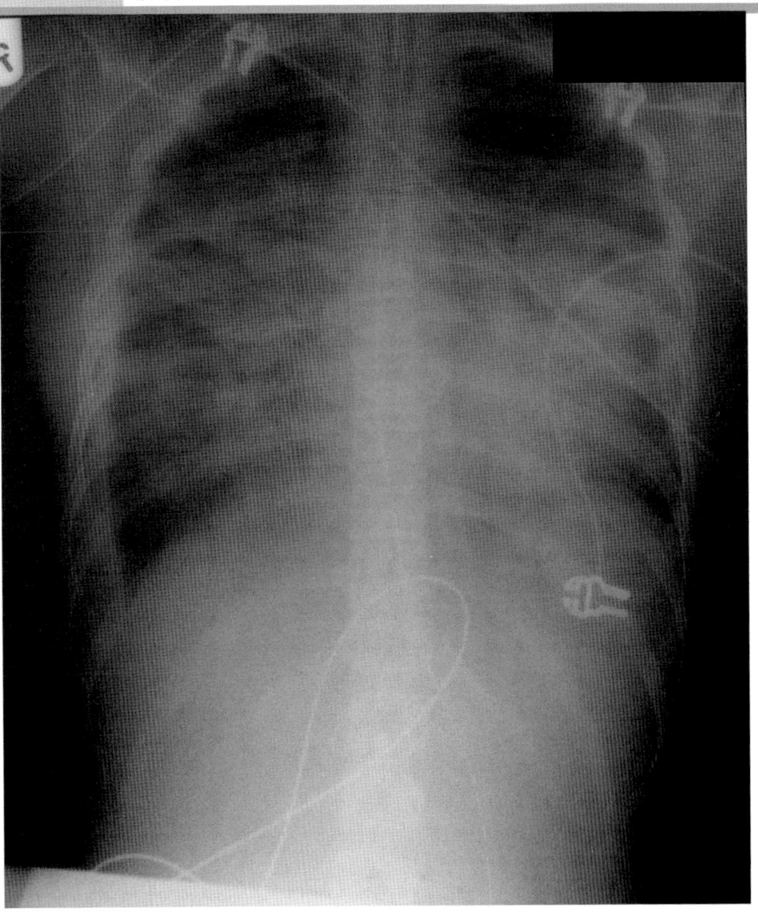

Initial impression

Bilateral white lungs.

Interpretation

The film confirms the correct siting of the endotracheal and nasogastric tubes. The tip of the endotracheal tube should be at least 2 cm from the carina to avoid intubation of the main bronchus. There are ECG leads on the patient.

Close examination of the whiteness shows an air bronchogram with the airways showing up as dark structures against the white background. There are also bilateral pleural effusions. Patients on a ventilator are generally imaged supine. You will notice how the appearance of these effusions is very different to that on an erect film. When the patient is supine the fluid will not accumulate at the lung bases. In this film the fluid lies laterally and tracks into the fissure.

This widespread consolidation and bilateral pleural effusions could be due to an overwhelming pneumonia, but in this case this was caused by an idiopathic toxic effect of the chemotherapy.

SUMMARY

Widespread consolidation and bilateral pleural effusions.

CXR 21

This 67-year-old man was admitted with a chest infection. He initially responded to antibiotic treatment but became more unwell with swinging fevers. If you look carefully at the upper margin of the abnormal area on this film there is an air/fluid level. What are the potential causes of this?

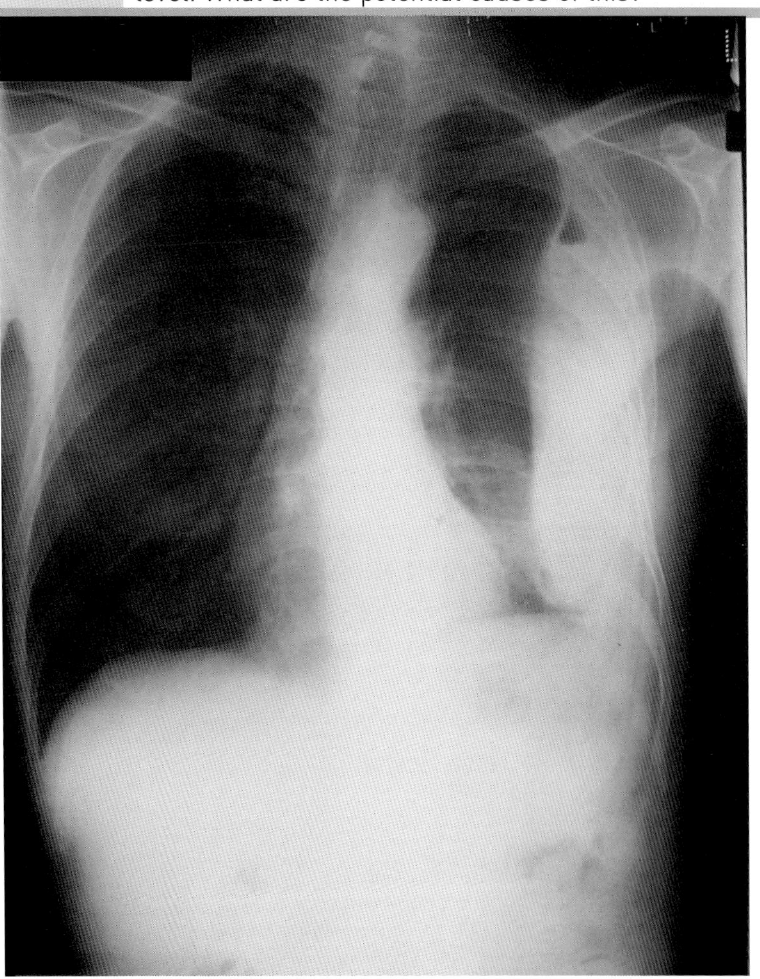

Initial assessment

Abnormal white density over the lateral edge of the left lung.

Interpretation

This density is very peripheral, and is parallel to the chest wall. These appearances are in keeping with a pleural collection. A simple pleural collection will generally remain free within the pleural space and move to the dependent areas, i.e. the lower part of the chest, with gravity. In this case, however, the fluid is no longer free, and has been walled away (this is likely to have happened when the patient was lying down) and a fibroblastic response has occurred, walling off an infected pleural collection. The potential causes for an air/fluid level within this include the presence of a gas-forming organism, a bronchopleural fistula, or iatrogenic – air may have been introduced into the chest during a diagnostic or therapeutic aspiration.

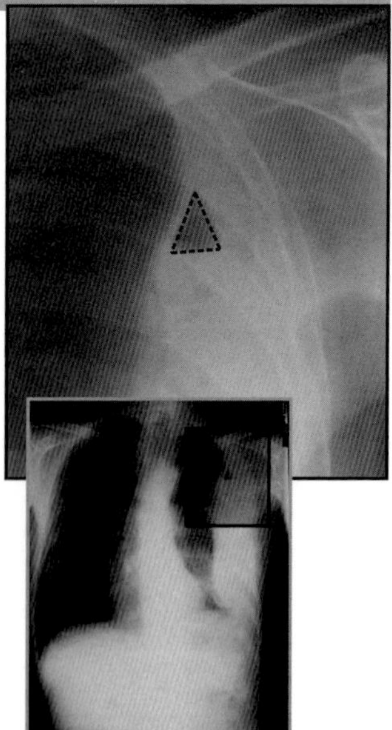

SUMMARY

Complex pleural collection in the periphery of the left hemithorax.

CXR 22

A 65-year-old woman had a cardiorespiratory arrest on the ward and was successfully resuscitated from ventricular fibrillation. This was the post arrest film. What action do you need to take?

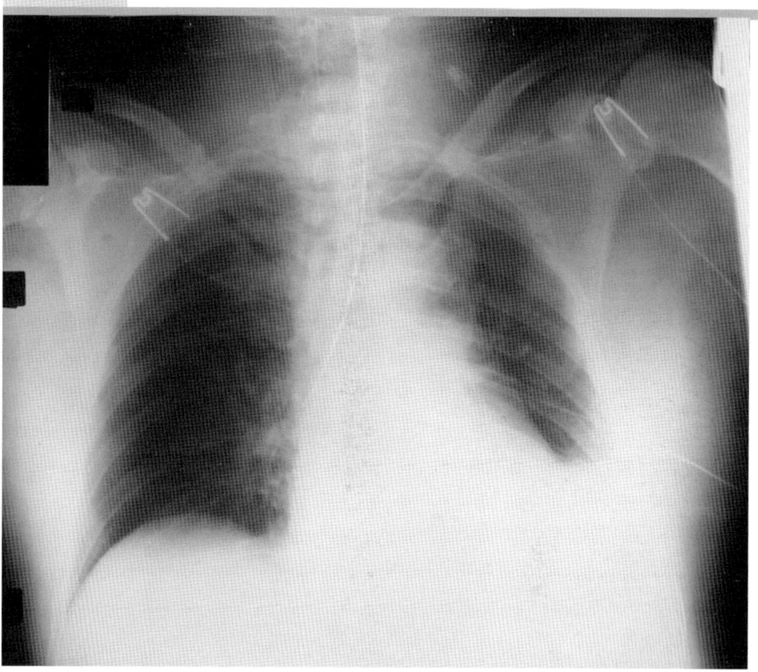

Initial assessment

Abnormal white lung on the left side.

Interpretation

The left hemidiaphragm is not clearly seen; there is increased whiteness at the left lung base and the mediastinum is swung towards the left side. This could be due to collapse of the left lung or a pneumothorax on the right, pushing the mediastinum to the left. It is possible that one of these has developed as a complication of insertion of one of the tubes or lines seen on this film.

You need to check the positions of the tubes and lines in this patient. The right jugular line is not very far into the vessel, but there is no evidence of there being a right pneumothorax as a cause for the mediastinal shift. There is a nasogastric tube in place and the tip of this cannot be seen, but it remains central in the lower chest and therefore is within the oesophagus. The endotracheal tube lies to the left of the midline and this reflects the left-sided volume loss in the lung. The tip of the endotracheal tube, however, lies within the proximal right main bronchus. This means that the left chest is not ventilated and gases within the lung are being reabsorbed, leading to volume loss and partial collapse of the left lung. You need to withdraw the tube by 3–5 cm to re-inflate the left lung.

SUMMARY

Endotracheal tube in right main bronchus. The tube needs to be withdrawn by 3–5 cm.

CXR 23

This elderly woman collapsed in the out-patient clinic and was resuscitated by the crash team. After an initial recovery and a failed attempt at inserting a central line, she deteriorated again and this film was taken. What immediate action would you take?

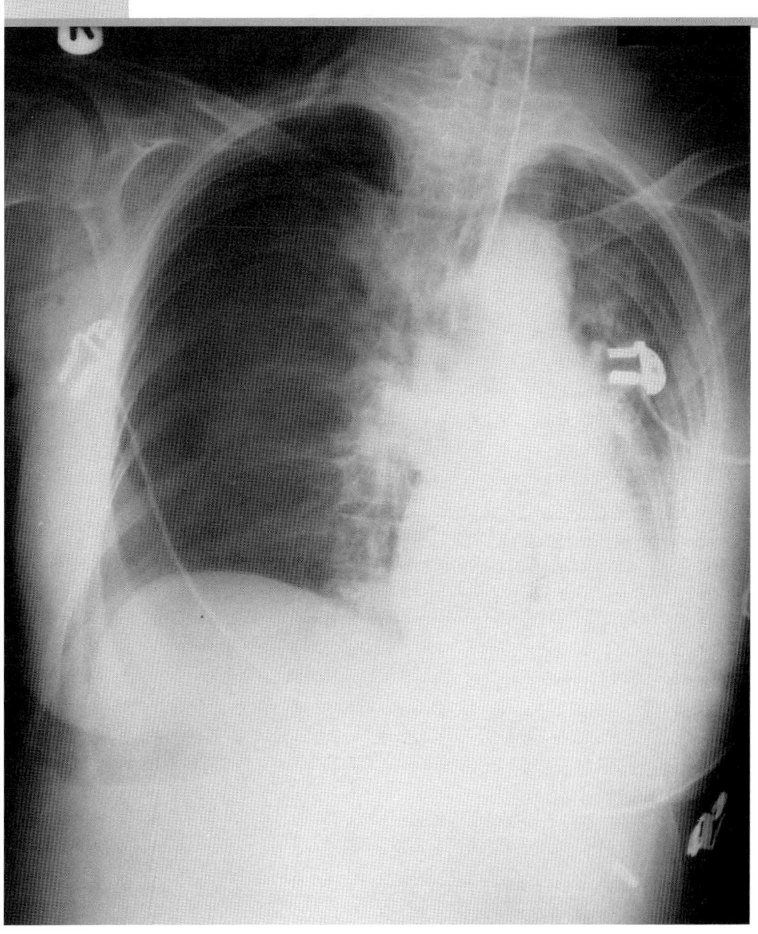

Initial impression

Abnormal black right lung.

Interpretation

The right lung is abnormally black. The patient is obviously deteriorating rapidly and you must first look for a pneumothorax, as this would be a treatable cause of her deterioration. Look for a lung edge, which in this film can be seen on the right side. Look also for a shift of the mediastinum, which, in a tension pneumothorax, will be pushed away from the area of black lung. The film here is slightly rotated, as assessed by looking at the clavicles, but even allowing for this the mediastinum is shifted, along with the heart, into the left side of the chest. The presence of the endotracheal tube helps to indicate that there is significant mediastinal shift.

On the full survey of the film, some air in the soft tissues over the right supraclavicular area can be seen. This would suggest that the pneumothorax was caused by the attempt at central line insertion on this side.

There is a subtle sign associated with this pneumothorax. Look at the area under the right diaphragm. You can see a curved line sloping downwards from the right heart border to the lateral chest wall. This is the posterior portion of the diaphragm which has been inverted because of the tension pneumothorax. In a supine patient this may be the only feature of a pneumothorax.

SUMMARY

Iatrogenic pneumothorax. A chest drain needs to be inserted immediately.

CXR 24

This 69-year-old woman who is known to have lung cancer was seen in the follow-up clinic where she reported an increase in breathlessness. What is the cause of her symptoms?

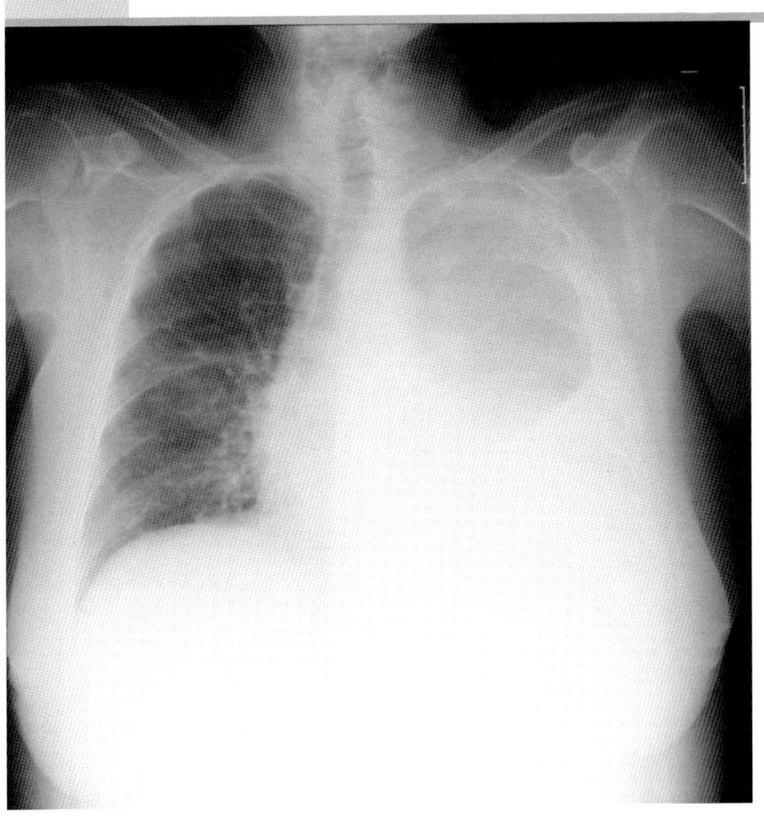

Initial impression

White left lung.

Interpretation

First note that the film is a little rotated – the heads of the clavicles are not equidistant from the spinous processes.

There are two distinct areas of whiteness. The first is a 'white out' of the lower left chest where the diaphragms and all the lung markings are obscured. This area of whiteness tracks around the lateral chest wall and even surrounds the lung at the apex. This is a pleural effusion.

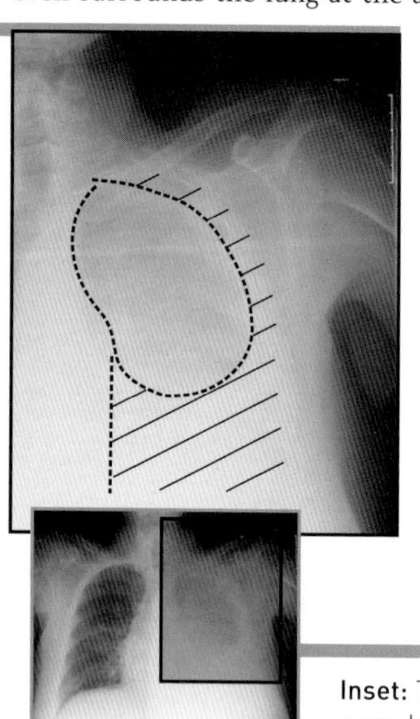

The second area of whiteness is over the left upper lung field and has a different appearance. If you examine this area carefully you will see a generalized increase in shadowing which does not obscure the bronchial or vascular markings. This is called ground glass shadowing. Remember that on a plain X-ray the commonest cause will be a pleural effusion.

Inset: The hatched area is the completely white area due to fluid. This surrounds the greyer area of ground-glass shadowing, where some underlying air-filled lung can still be identified.

SUMMARY

Pleural effusion.

CXR 25

This 74-year-old retired demolition worker presented to his GP with exertional breathlessness. The GP ordered this film. What does it show?

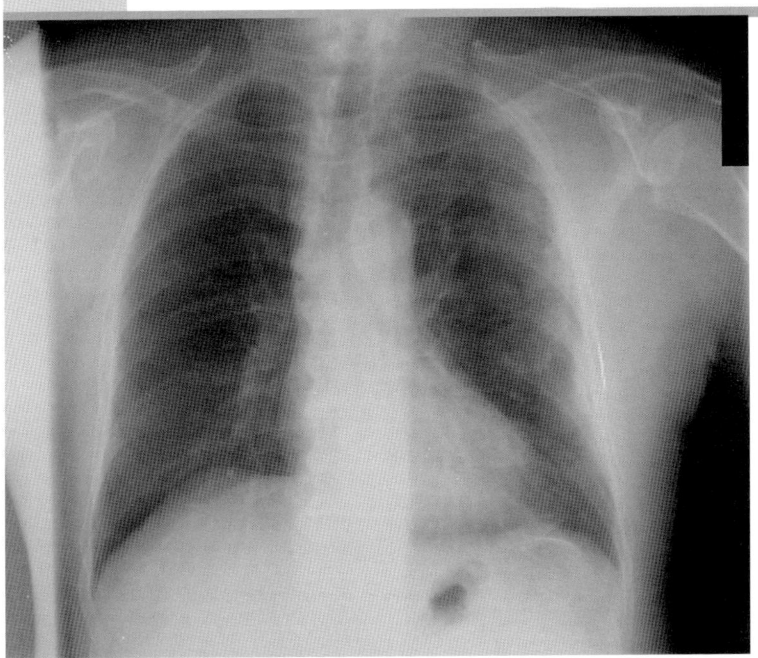

Initial impression

White lung shadows.

Interpretation

Initial inspection of the lung fields shows a number of dense white shadows. You need to look at the nature of these shadows. The shadows are irregularly shaped and have a map-like appearance due to calcification within them. They are sometimes said to have a holly leaf appearance. This is typical of pleural plaques that are usually caused by asbestos exposure. Look for other signs of pleural disease due to asbestos exposure. If you look at the edge of the lung fields you will see that the pleura is much thicker than usual, especially on the left. You can tell this because, unusually, you can see it very clearly. If you also look at the apex of the left diaphragm you will see an area of calcification, which is another consequence of asbestos exposure.

Now you have characterized the nature of the shadows, you need to look at their distribution. These shadows are all orientated along the anterior ends of the ribs, which would be common with asbestos plaques. However, the unilateral nature of the plaques is unusual for asbestos related plaques.

Causes of pleural change with calcification include asbestos exposure, tuberculosis and trauma with haemothorax. In this case the pleural thickening was due to asbestos related pleural disease.

SUMMARY

Pleural plaques.

CXR 26

What is the cause of this 57-year-old woman's breathlessness?

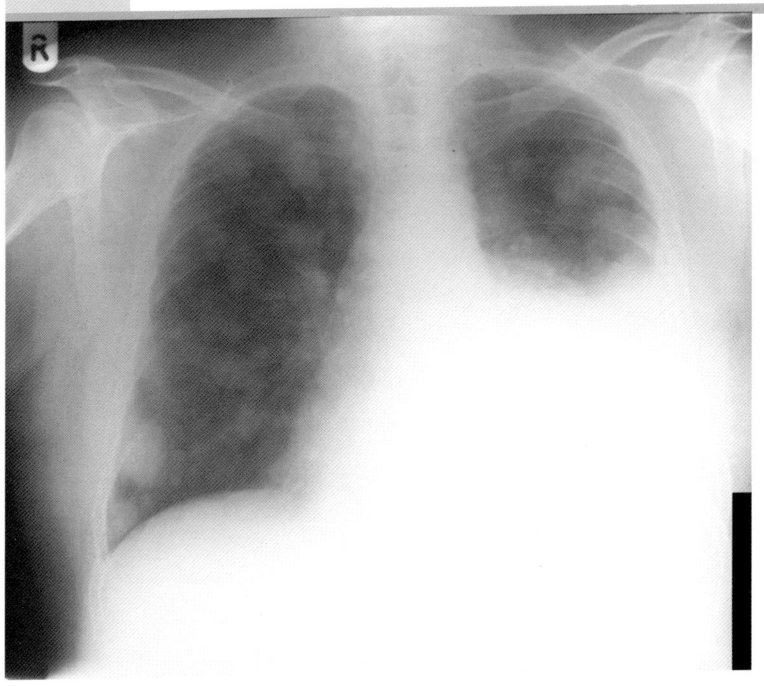

Initial impression

White left lung.

Interpretation

There is an obvious area of whiteness in the left lung. This is homogeneous in nature and has a well-defined upper edge and a meniscus – it is a pleural effusion.

Once you have diagnosed a pleural effusion you need to look for any clues as to the cause. Look carefully at the lung fields in this film. You can see numerous white nodules throughout both the right and left lungs. Look at the features of these nodules. They are all different sizes and densities and most have an irregular, lobulated appearance. The variation in size and density, and the lobulated appearance of some of the nodules would suggest that they are pulmonary metastases. The pleural effusion is likely to be caused by malignancy.

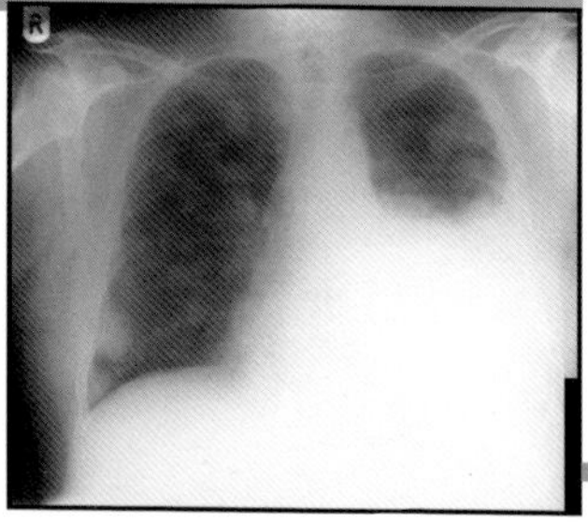

Above: Metastases are usually spread via the blood stream and, as in this case, when there are multiple metastases, they tend to be predominantly peripheral and basal.

SUMMARY

Malignant pleural effusion with pulmonary metastases.

CXR 27

This patient's PA film revealed an abnormality in the left lung field, shown here in the lateral. What abnormality is present on this lateral film, and where is it located?

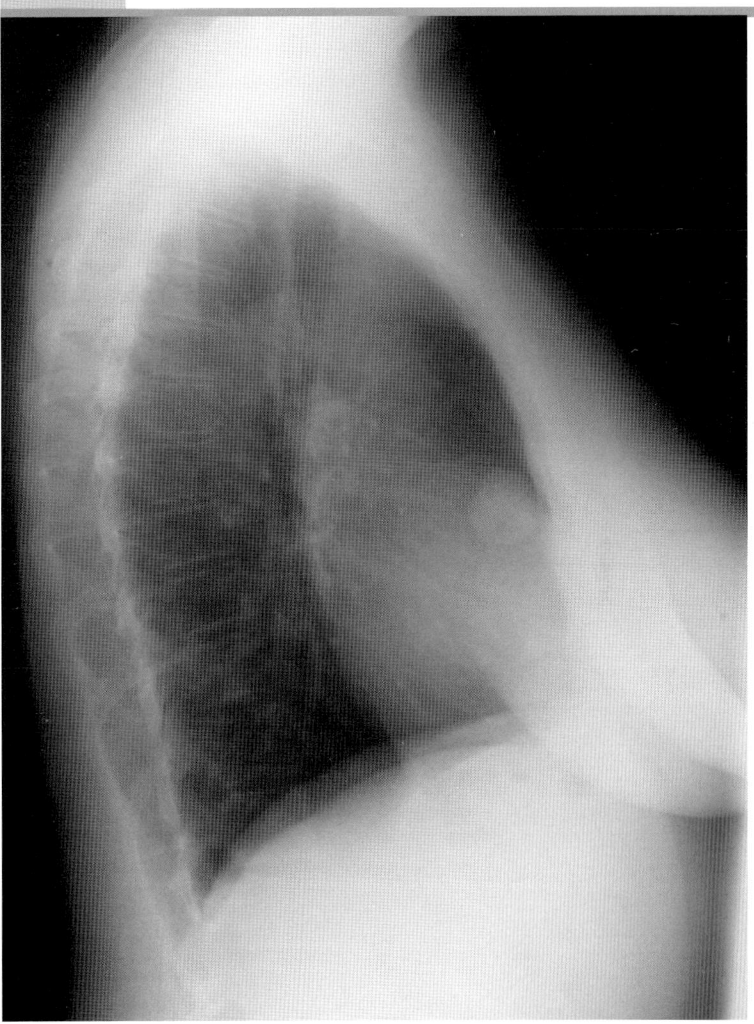

Initial impression

Coin lesion.

Interpretation

A coin lesion can be seen on this lateral film. The lesion lies very anteriorly – it is certainly anterior to the oblique fissure and it therefore lies in the left upper lobe. Peripheral lung nodules are less likely to be seen at bronchoscopy and a diagnosis can be obtained by biopsy under fluoroscopic or CT guidance.

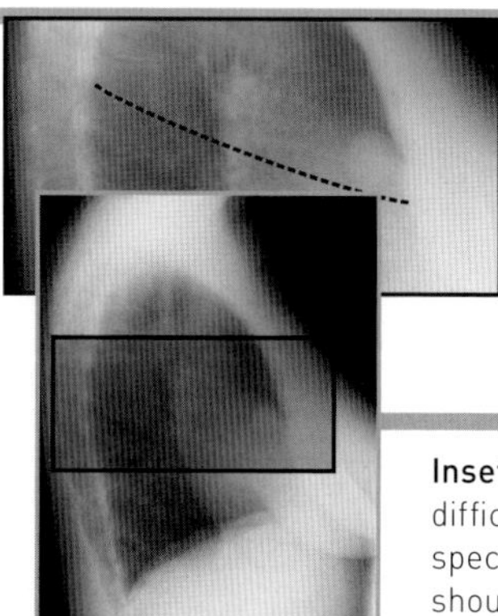

Inset: The oblique fissure may sometimes be difficult to identify on the lateral view. In order to specify that this coin lesion is in the upper lobe you should be aware that the normal fissures will start posteriorly at around the level of T6, then pass down to the diaphragm about one quarter of the way back from the anterior chest wall.

SUMMARY

Left upper lobe coin lesion.

CXR 28

This 79-year-old man complained of cough and right-sided chest pain. In the light of the film, what questions would you ask the patient?

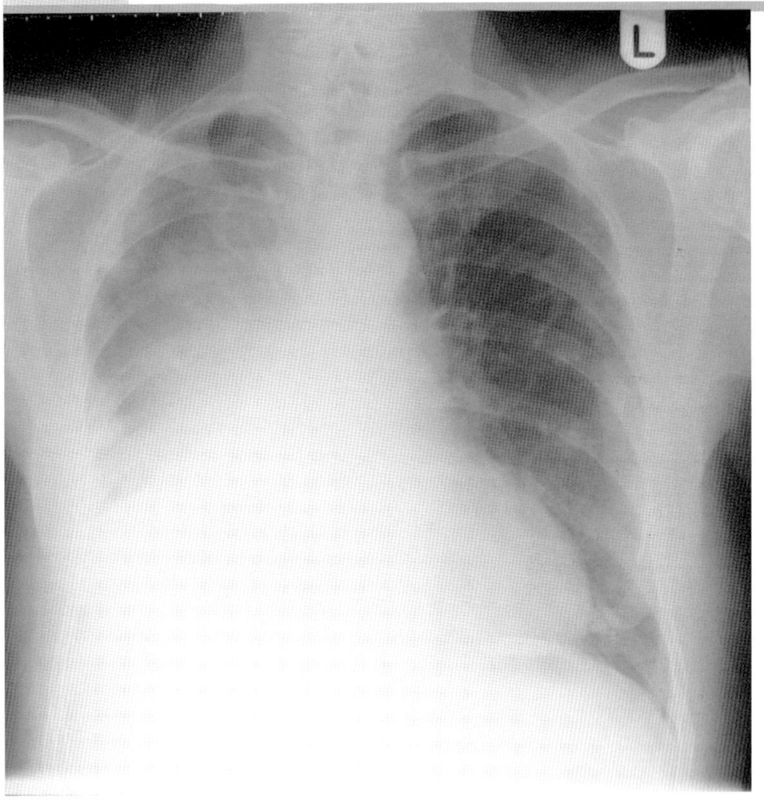

Initial impression

Complicated film with areas of whiteness in the right lung and scattered areas of whiteness in the left lung.

Interpretation

This is a complicated film that contains a number of abnormalities. The most obvious is the area of whiteness at the base of the right lung, which is in continuity with the mediastinal shadow. Examine this area carefully. Look at the nature of the whiteness. It is homogeneous, which goes against consolidation, but would be consistent with lung collapse or an effusion. The mediastinum is central, which goes against there being a large area of collapse. It is an effusion.

There are clues on the film as to the cause of the effusion: there are multiple areas of whiteness over the left lung field. Look at the distribution; they run along the line of the border of the ribs. This distribution suggests they are pleural plaques. This diagnosis is supported by the presence of calcification in some of these areas, and a plaque over the curvature of the left hemidiaphragm which is also calcified.

You need to ask the patient whether they have had any exposure to asbestos.

There are many complications of asbestos exposure: benign pleural plaques, extensive pleural thickening that can impair ventilation, malignant mesothelioma, or interstitial lung fibrosis known as asbestosis. The presence of a large effusion in this patient may indicate an underlying mesothelioma. A pleural biopsy and drainage of the fluid were performed, which unfortunately confirmed this diagnosis. Mesothelioma has a very poor prognosis.

SUMMARY

Pleural plaques and pleural effusion due to mesothelioma. The patient needs to be asked about asbestos exposure.

CXR 29

This 32-year-old man presented with a 5-day history of cough and left-sided chest pain. What is the abnormality on the film?

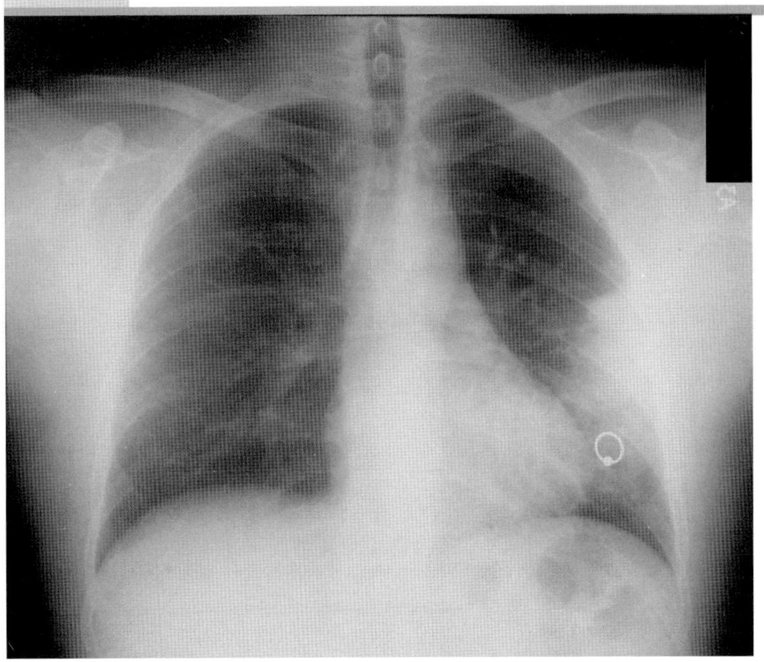

Initial impression

There is a nipple ring. Abnormal white lung in the periphery of the left lung.

Interpretation

The muscles of the shoulder girdle increase the whiteness around the chest in the upper to mid zones. This can be very noticeable in people who do a lot of manual work, or training at the gymnasium. This can make interpretation of these areas difficult, and abnormalities may be overlooked. Usually the changes are fairly symmetrical. On this film, there is a triangular shaped wedge of increased density in the left mid zone. This is away from the heart border, so does not involve the lingular lobe. It could, however, involve the upper or lower lobe, and without a lateral film you cannot localize the abnormality very specifically.

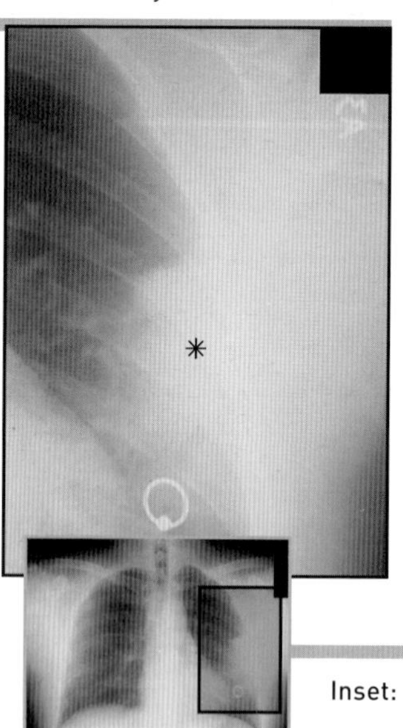

There is no obvious basal left-sided pleural effusion.

This is an isolated focus of triangular shaped consolidation. The differential would include infection. The history and film, however, could also fit a pulmonary embolism.

A ventilation perfusion study produced a low probability of pulmonary embolism, and the patient was treated for a community acquired pneumonia. He responded quickly, and the follow-up film was normal.

Inset: *Area of peripheral consolidation.

SUMMARY

Left mid zone consolidation.

CXR 30

This 53-year-old man came to hospital for a clinic appointment, and had this film taken before seeing his doctor. What relevant history does he have?

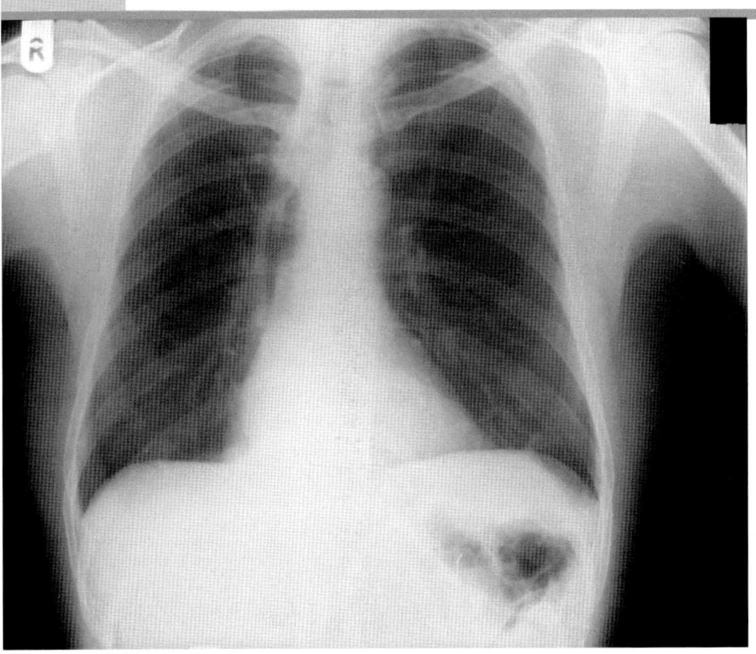

Initial impression

Abnormal mediastinum.

Interpretation

The film is not rotated. The right side of the mediastinum is abnormal. The mid portion of the mediastinum is involved and there is an abnormal dark band with a white outer margin. The trachea can be seen separately.

The majority of abnormal appearances of the mediastinum cause a white density. The presence here of a dark band limits the differential and causes would include air around the mediastinum (pneumomediastinum), which would have only a very thin white line around the outer margin. This thicker line suggests a structural wall, such as the wall of an abnormally dilated oesophagus. If, however, you look closely at the film, there is a clip visible under the left side of the diaphragm. This indicates previous surgery.

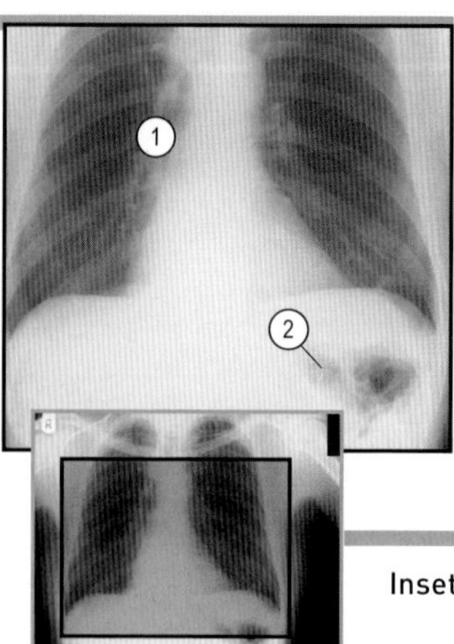

The relevant history here is of an oesophagectomy, and gastric pull-up, a procedure performed for oesophageal malignancy. On this occasion an abdominal approach was used and there has not been a thoracotomy.

Inset: 1. Wall of gastric pull-up. 2. Surgical clip.

SUMMARY

Post-oesophagectomy.

CXR 31

This 24-year-old man had been extremely unwell for 4 weeks, with a swinging fever, loss of appetite, and weight loss. This is his film. What would be the next investigation?

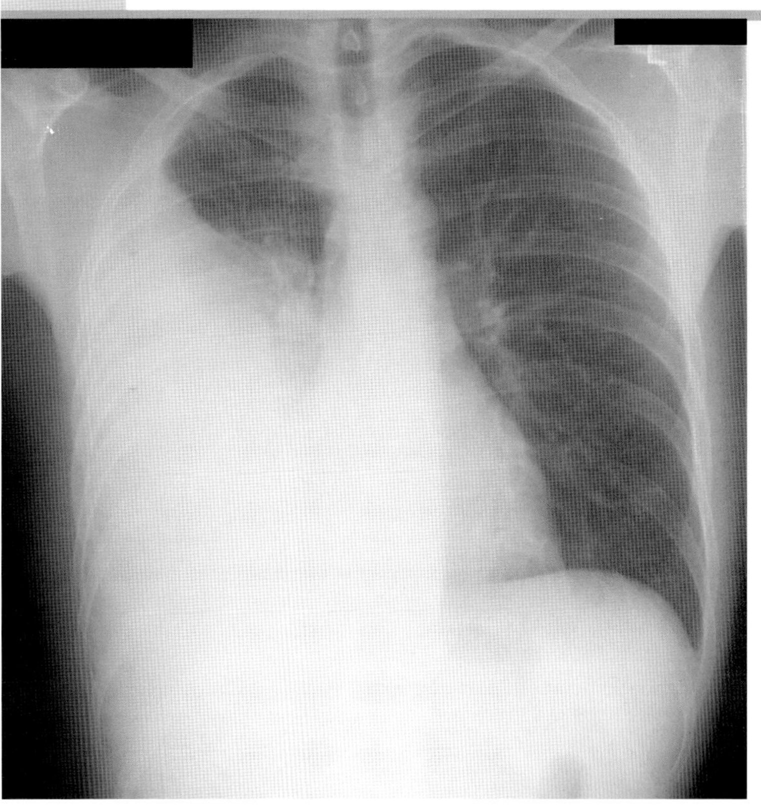

Initial impression

White right lung.

Interpretation

There is a large area of whiteness in the right lung field. The whiteness is homogeneous in nature and is due to a pleural effusion. Look at the upper border. Although you may expect a single white line to demarcate the upper border of an effusion, remember that the lung is a three-dimensional structure. The lower part of the effusion looks a lot denser; here the underlying lung is compressed by a larger volume of fluid. The upper edge of the effusion is less white and there is less fluid here, but it is surrounding aerated lung. This is why you can see lung markings through the fluid. It is because of the two densities of fluid that the upper border appears to have a double edge.

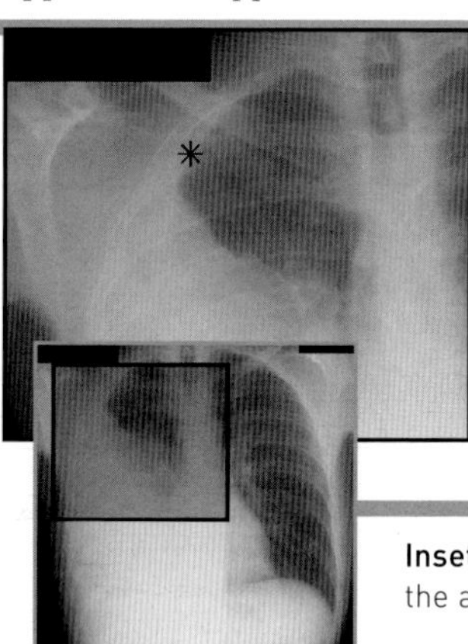

Inset: Large effusions tend to run up and around the apex of the lung.*

SUMMARY

Right pleural effusion. Aspiration of this effusion would be the next investigation, and samples should be sent for microbiology, cytology and chemistry. An empyema is likely to be the diagnosis in view of the radiological and clinical features.

CXR 32

This 34-year-old man noticed some swelling over his shoulder. His GP noted that he had lymphadenopathy in the supraclavicular and axillary regions and elicited a history of weight loss, pruritus and night sweats. This is his film. What is the most likely diagnosis?

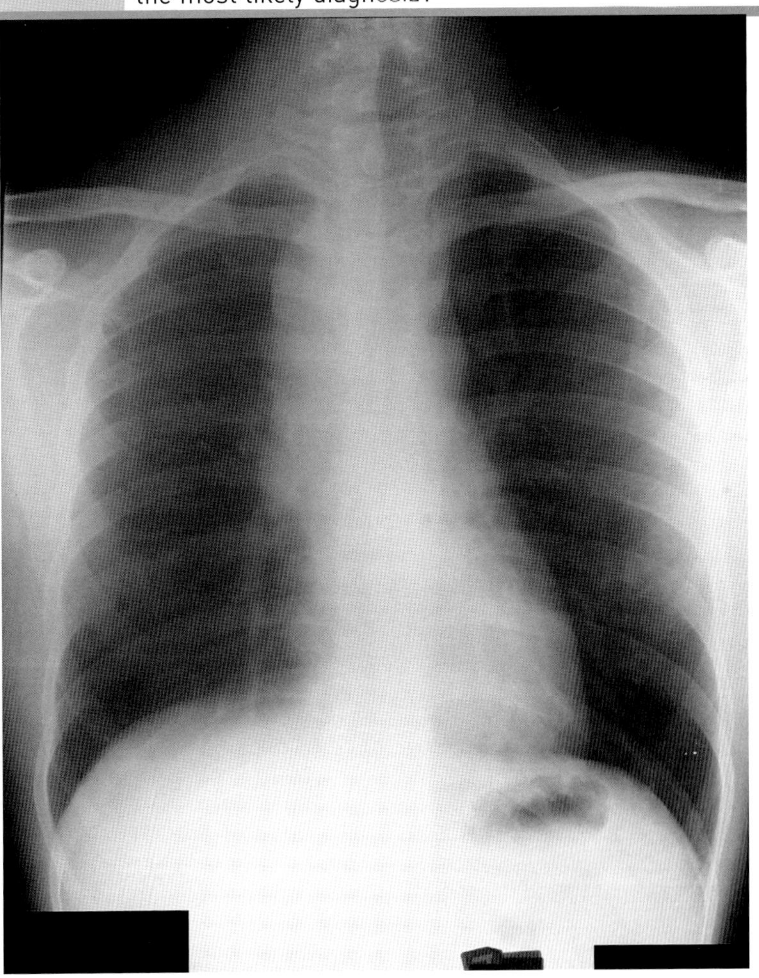

Initial impression

Abnormal area of whiteness to the right of the mediastinum.

Interpretation

There is not usually any density seen to the right side of the trachea from the level of the head of the clavicles to the carina, and the white edge of the trachea should always be under 2–3 mm on an erect film. On this film you can see a dense white, homogeneous shadow in this area. The upper border of the right hilum is not visible because this mass overlies it. The position of the whiteness, closely bound to the mediastinum and merging with the hilum, suggests that this is an enlarged mediastinal structure. Look at the trachea; it has been pushed to the left by this mass.

Look at the soft tissues over the shoulders. There is a fullness and increased density of the soft tissue in the right supraclavicular area (where the GP felt lymph nodes). The combination of mediastinal and supraclavicular soft tissue enlargement would be in keeping with the clinical picture of diffuse lymphadenopathy.

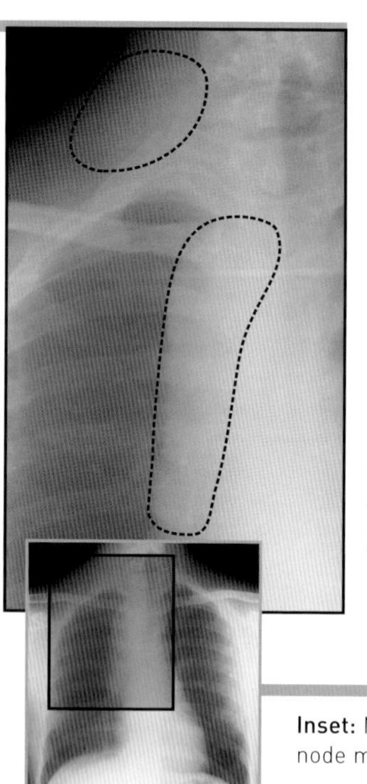

Inset: Mediastinal and right supraclavicular lymph node masses.

SUMMARY

Mediastinal and right supraclavicular lymphadenopathy, most likely due to Hodgkin's lymphoma. This was confirmed at biopsy.

CXR 33

This is the film of a 48-year-old local government officer who is under follow-up in the cardiology clinic. What is the likely underlying abnormality?

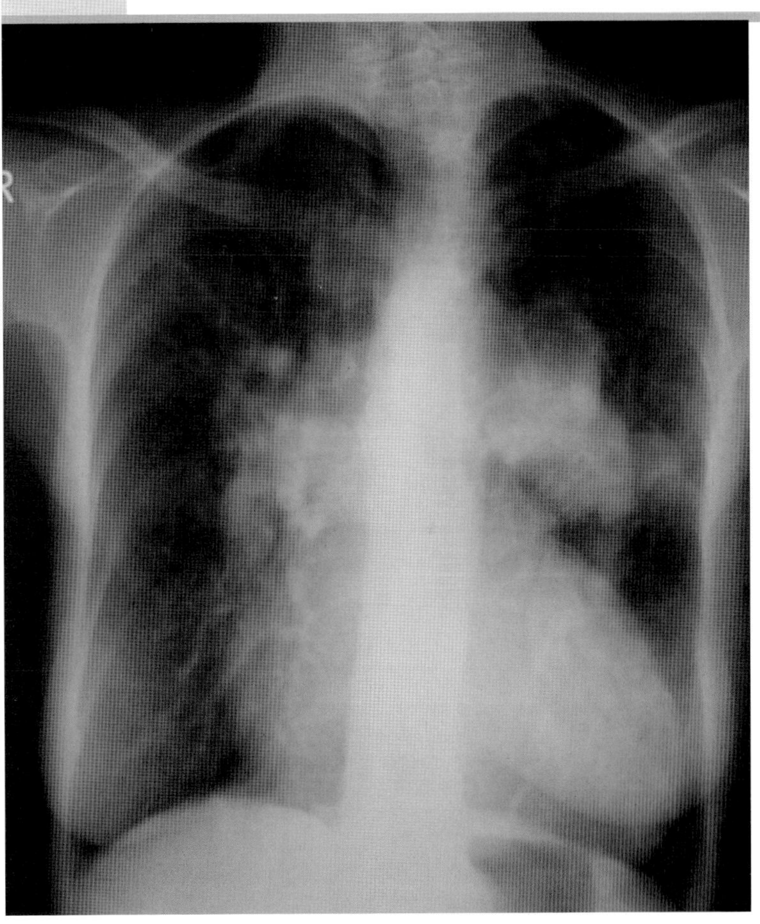

Initial impression

Abnormal white shadowing at the hila.

Interpretation

Bilateral white shadows at the hila could be due to lymph node enlargement, or enlarged pulmonary arteries. The shadows are unlikely to be due to masses in front of or behind the hila, as they are bilateral. These white shadows give off branches indicating they are enlarged pulmonary arteries. The vessels show 'pruning', a term that means that they end abruptly, rather than gradually tapering out towards the periphery of the lung. Causes for enlargement would include chronic thrombo-embolic disease, or cardiac disease. Pulmonary emboli when chronic cause a sustained rise in pulmonary artery pressure and this will frequently produce vessel enlargement. Cardiac causes may lead to a pressure or a volume load on the circulation.

Look carefully at the heart, which is enlarged in this case, implying a cardiac cause. This lady has a ventricular septal defect with flow from the left to right ventricle. This has led to both a volume and a pressure load on the pulmonary arteries.

SUMMARY

Cardiac shunt.

CXR 34

This 71-year-old man is brought to hospital by ambulance following a collapse in the street. What does this film show?

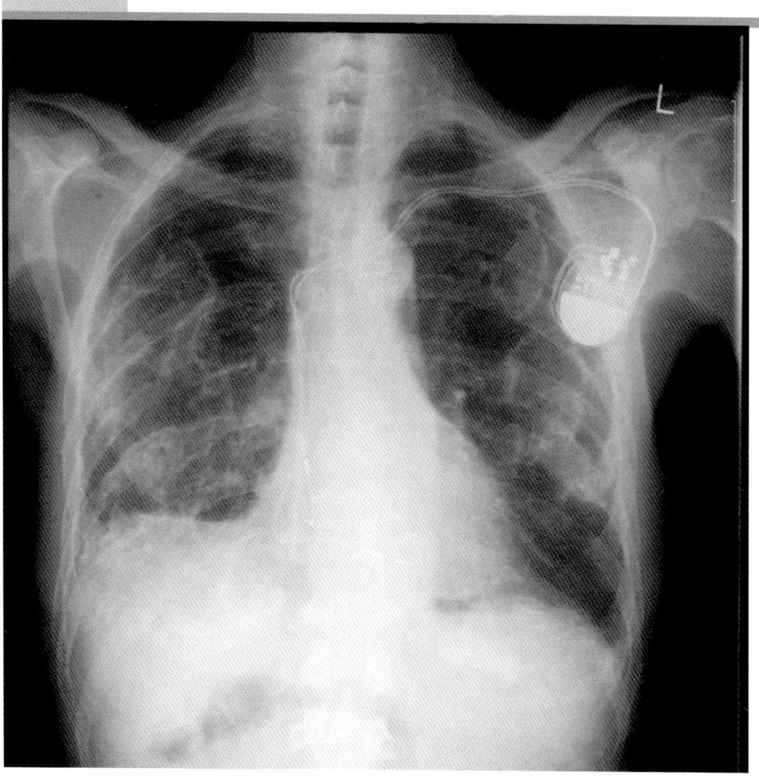

Initial impression

Abnormal white lung on both sides. In addition there is a metal density box and wires over the left upper chest.

Interpretation

There are prominent areas of whiteness over both sides of the chest. The marked density indicates that they are calcified. They are not limited by the lobar boundaries and seem to lie along the axis of the ribs in some areas. The margins are well defined but irregular – the so-called holly leaf appearance. These are pleural plaques.

The metal density box in the upper zone is a permanent pacemaker. There are two wires leading from this, passing along the subclavian vein, brachiocephalic vein, and into the superior vena cava, with one lead in the right atrium and the other in the right ventricle. Further wires noted over the sternum indicate previous cardiac surgery.

In a patient with a collapse and a pacemaker in situ, it is important to check that the pacemaker is working correctly. In this patient there was a malfunction.

The pleural plaques are an incidental finding.

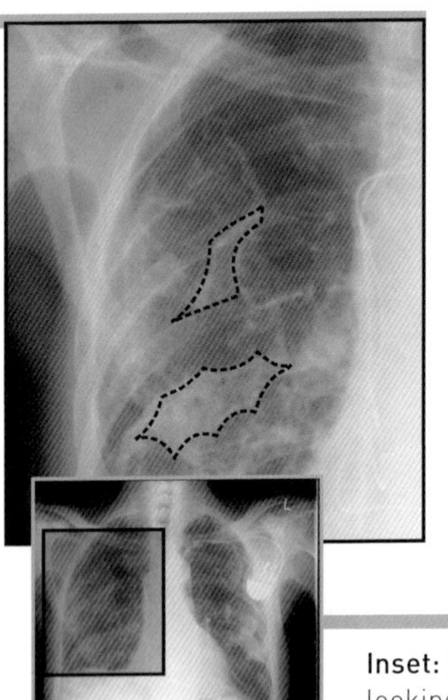

Inset: Pleural plaques are classically described as looking like a holly leaf.

SUMMARY

Permanent dual chamber pacemaker. Pleural plaques.

CXR 35

This is the film of a 20-year-old law student who is on immunosuppression following a renal transplant. What diagnoses could the film suggest?

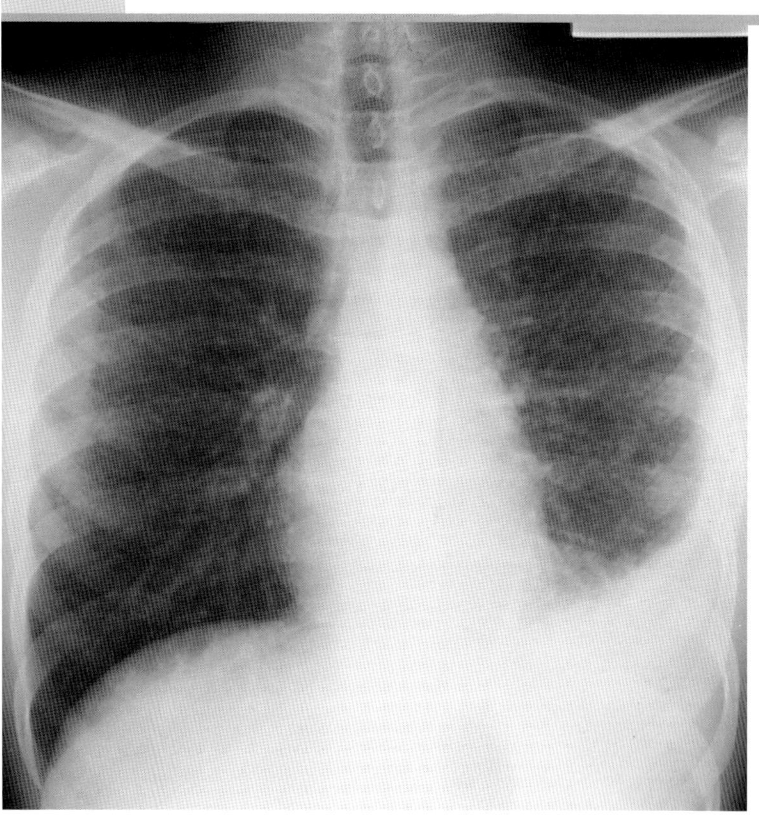

Initial impression

Multiple small white nodules in both lungs and abnormal whiteness at the left lung base.

Interpretation

There are multiple small rounded densities of roughly the same size scattered through both lungs. This pattern of small nodules is called 'miliary'. No hila or mediastinal adenopathy can be seen.

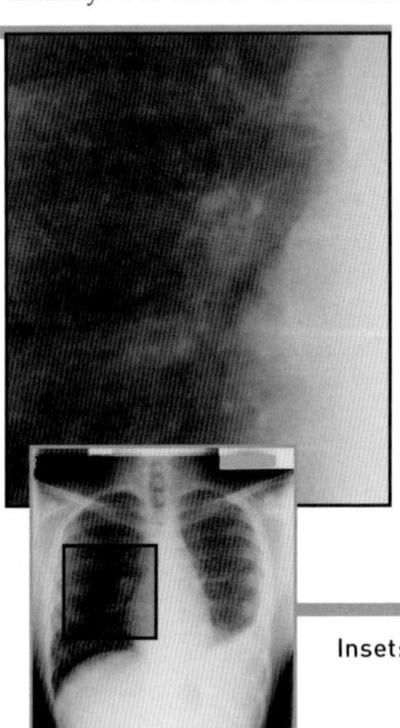

This pattern is recognized in the blood-borne spread of tuberculosis, in either a young child or a patient with an abnormal immune system. Other potential causes for this pattern would include sarcoidosis, metastases or silicosis, an occupational lung disease from exposure to silica dust.

In this clinical setting, miliary tuberculosis needs to be excluded.

Inset: Multifocal soft nodules.

SUMMARY

Miliary tuberculosis with a left pleural effusion. The differential would include sarcoidosis, metastases and, with an appropriate clinical history, silicosis.

CXR 36

This 75-year-old woman went to see her GP following two episodes of haemoptysis. She smoked 15 cigarettes per day. What would be the next appropriate investigations?

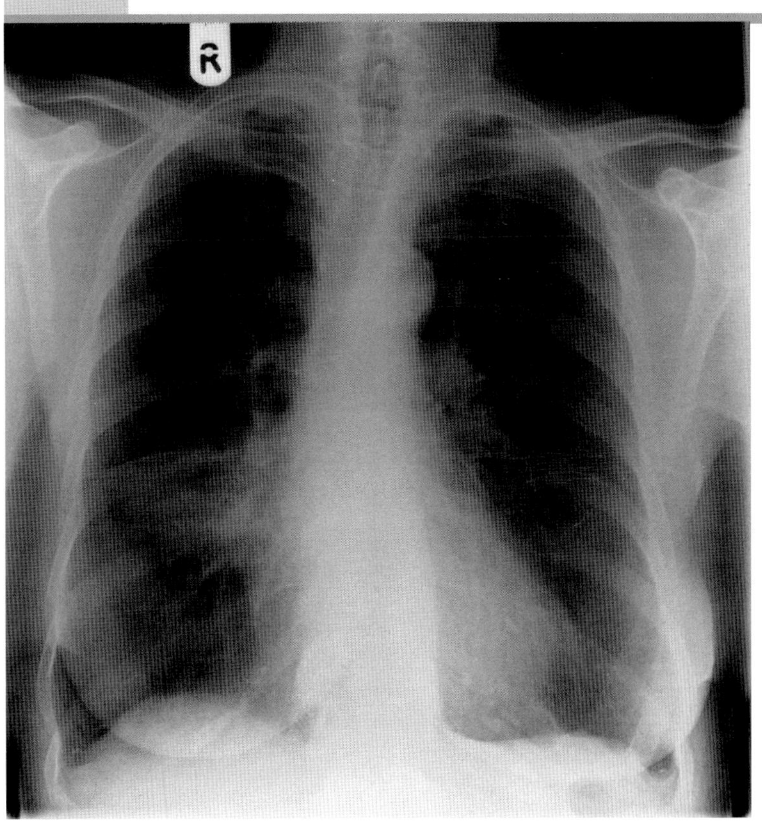

Initial impression

Area of whiteness in the right lung.

Interpretation

There is a hazy shadowing in the right mid zone and the mediastinal border at this level is obscured. This is the typical appearance of right middle lobe collapse. This can be difficult to spot and other features to look for, although not present on this film, are a raised right hemidiaphragm and downward displacement of the horizontal fissure. Right middle lobe collapse is often easier to spot on a lateral film.

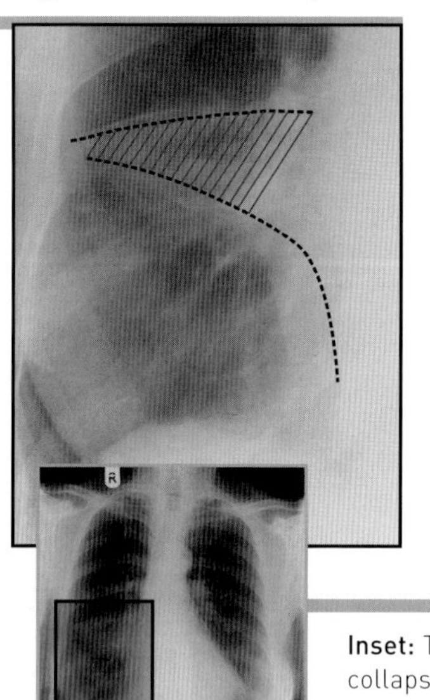

This woman could have a malignant lesion in the middle lobe bronchus causing the haemoptysis and middle lobe collapse, though the differential diagnosis would include an inhaled foreign body or pneumonia with associated lung collapse. The next investigations would be fibreoptic bronchoscopy and a CT scan.

Inset: Typical outline of a right middle lobe collapse.

SUMMARY

Right middle lobe collapse. The next investigations would be a fibreoptic bronchoscopy and CT scanning.

CXR 37

This 53-year-old shop worker has noticed increasing breathlessness over the last 6 months, associated with a dry cough. What is the diagnosis and what would you expect to find on examination?

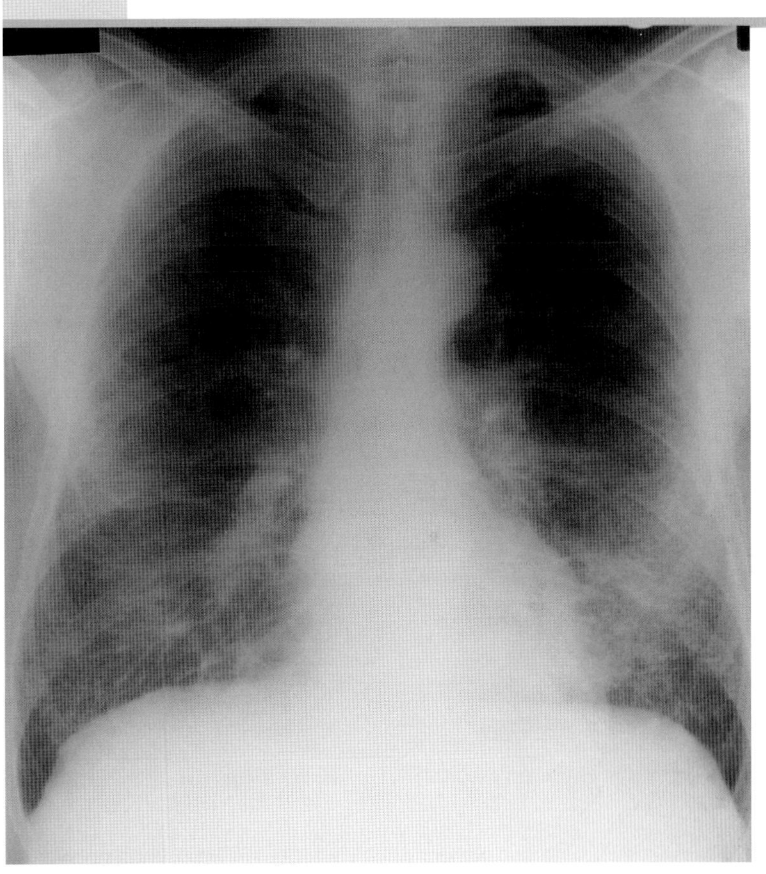

Initial impression

Bilateral basal white lung.

Interpretation

There is a whiteness in the lower zones of both lungs. You need to decide on the nature of this whiteness. It is not homogeneous so will not be lung collapse or bilateral pleural effusions. The main possibilities would be consolidation, pulmonary oedema, metastases or an interstitial fibrosis. Look carefully at the nature of the shadowing. Consolidation causes an air bronchogram, pulmonary oedema tends to have a perihilar distribution, and metastases are usually discrete small round nodules. The shadowing here does not have these appearances. Fibrosis causes a series of criss-crossing lines that will appear like a mesh over the lung and in later stages like a honeycomb. This is the appearance of the whiteness in this film. It is also useful to look at the margins of the diaphragm and heart border. In fibrotic lung disease they often look 'fluffy', a feature well demonstrated on this film, especially at the left heart border.

Other features are helpful in distinguishing pulmonary fibrosis from pulmonary oedema. In this film the heart size is normal, which would go against pulmonary oedema. Old films are useful since fibrosis is usually a chronic process and its presence in previous films would be very supportive of this diagnosis. Later on in the disease, pulmonary fibrosis can cause the lungs to shrink although this is not the case here.

This man went on to have a high resolution CT confirming a diagnosis of pulmonary fibrosis.

SUMMARY

Cryptogenic fibrosing alveolitis. On examination you would expect to hear fine, late inspiratory crackles.

CXR 38

This 43-year-old woman presented to her GP with a 10-day history of haemoptysis. On further questioning she admitted to a 3-month history of poor appetite and weight loss. How would you interpret the film and what investigation would you do next?

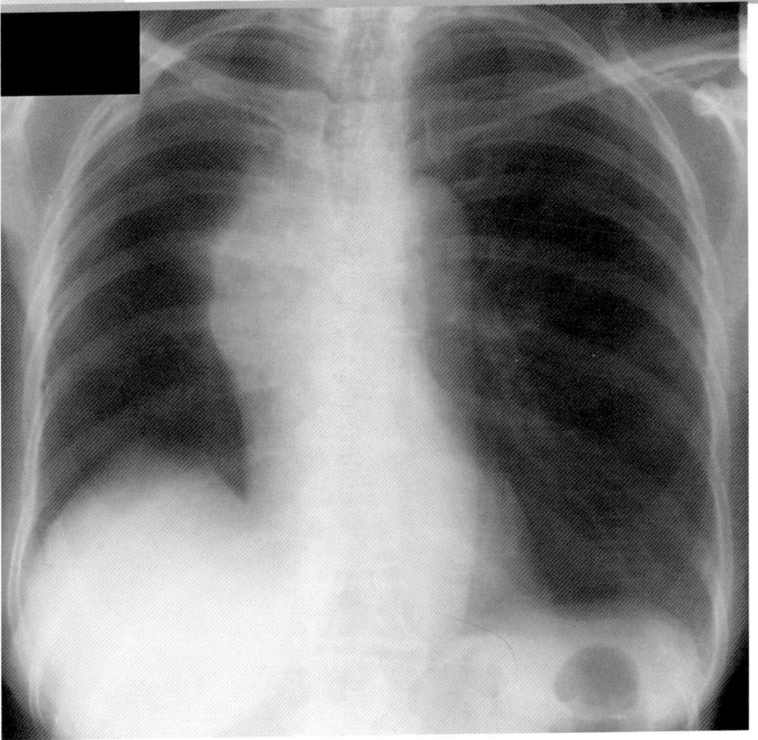

Initial impression

Abnormally shaped enlarged right hilum.

Interpretation

The obvious abnormality is the enlarged, abnormally shaped right hilum. This could be due to a mass in front of or behind the hilum, hilar lymph node enlargement or abnormally shaped hilar blood vessels. Look carefully at the shape of the enlarged area and at its edge. The area of enlargement is lobulated and the edge is not distinct. Careful examination shows the margin to be slightly blurred. The lobulated appearance and blurred edge would both go against a vascular cause for the enlargement since vascular shadows have a smooth distinct edge. Instead, these features suggest a tumour or enlarged lymph nodes with the blurred margins suggesting infiltration of the lung.

You should also look at the rest of the lung for additional clues. The right diaphragm is pulled up and there is deviation of the trachea to the right. This indicates collapse within the right lung. As the mass involves the lung and mediastinum, there is probably invasion into the right upper lobe bronchus, causing the collapse. Careful inspection of the lung fields shows there to be at least three small rounded nodules in the left lung. These would be consistent with pulmonary metastases and are further evidence that this is likely to be a malignancy.

SUMMARY

Primary lung cancer with right upper lobe collapse and pulmonary metastases. Further investigations would include CT scanning and fibreoptic bronchoscopy.

CXR 39

This 25-year-old telephone sales clerk was referred to the gastroenterology clinic for investigation of weight loss. She had no other symptoms. This film was taken at her first clinic visit and she was subsequently referred to the chest clinic. What does the film show?

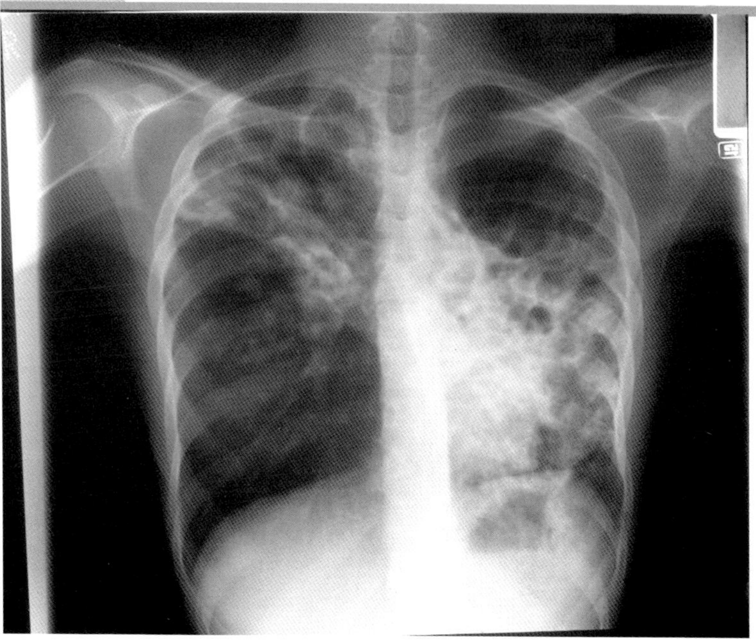

Initial impression

Abnormal areas of whiteness in the lungs.

Interpretation

There is extensive shadowing in both lung fields. Look at the nature of this shadowing. Within it there are multiple black areas. These are cavities and are most noticeable in the left lung. Look at the shadowing in the right upper zone. This has a streaky appearance, which is typical of pulmonary fibrosis. On the right side the shadowing is confined to the right upper lobe, whereas it is more widespread on the left. The combination of cavitating lung disease, co-existent fibrosis and a predilection for the upper lobes is very suggestive of tuberculosis. This woman's sputum was indeed positive for acid fast bacilli.

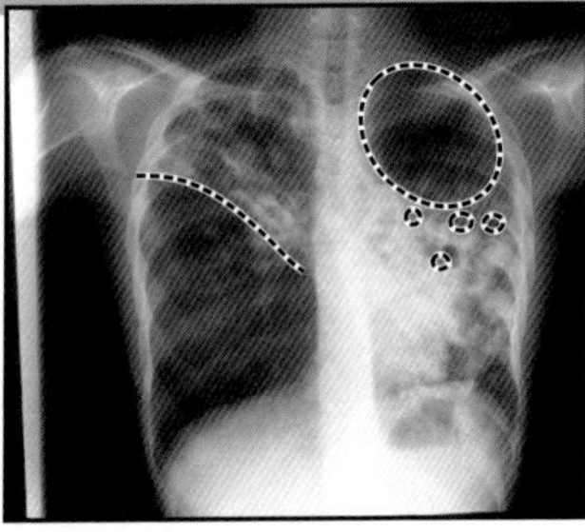

Above: Cavitation and lung distortion.

SUMMARY

Tuberculosis.

CXR 40

This 54-year-old fireman was admitted to hospital 3 days prior to this film, with severe upper abdominal pain. He was found to have a raised amylase and a diagnosis of acute pancreatitis was made, subsequently confirmed on CT scanning. This supine film was taken because the patient was complaining of increasing breathlessness. What is the cause of his increased breathlessness?

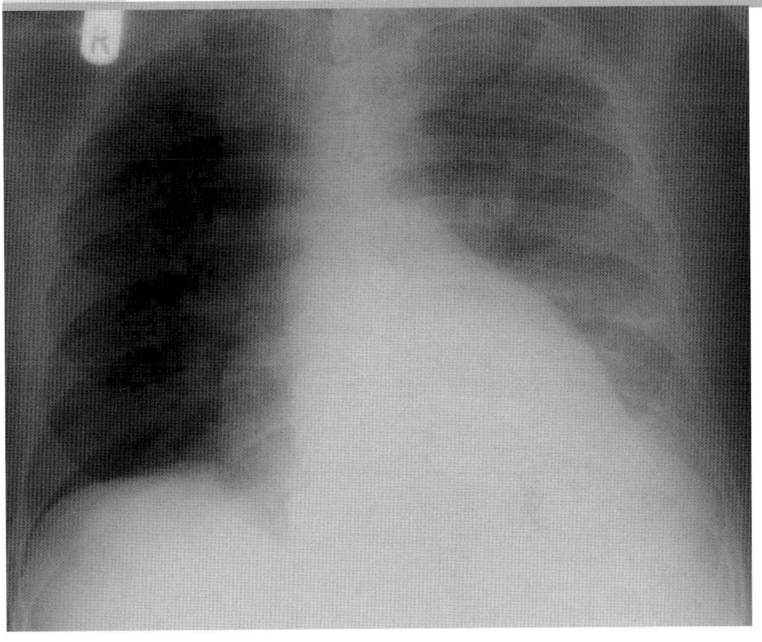

Initial impression

White left lung.

Interpretation

Be aware that this is a supine film and the film is slightly rotated to the left. The apices have been cropped from the study, which may indicate the need to repeat a film; it can be difficult to obtain a perfect film in a sick patient. There is a fairly homogeneous white shadow over the whole of the left lung field. Causes of whiteness would include lung collapse, consolidation and pleural fluid. You need to analyse each of these possibilities in turn.

Collapse: The film is slightly rotated but nevertheless it is clear that there is no tracheal shift to the left and the volume of the left lung appears normal. This would go against collapse as a cause of this appearance.

Consolidation: There is no air bronchogram visible, which would go against consolidation.

Pleural effusion: This does not have the typical appearance of a pleural effusion since there is no meniscus and no obvious fluid level. However, remember that the film has been taken with the patient supine, which means that the fluid will be distributed in the posterior pleural space and will not accumulate in the inferior part of the pleural space as it does when the patient is standing. In fact, with the patient lying supine, the fluid will tend to accumulate around the apices and track into the fissures, with some fluid at the base. Since the fluid is spread so diffusely it appears a lot less dense than when it is concentrated in the bases when the patient is sitting up or standing. This film shows the typical features of a pleural effusion on a supine film. There is diffuse low-density whiteness with increased whiteness in the apices and tracking along the fissures. The other lung field is normal and there is no mediastinal shift. This patient has a pleural effusion secondary to pancreatitis.

SUMMARY

Left-sided pleural effusion in a supine film.

CXR 41

This is the semi-erect film of a 67-year-old retired schoolteacher who was admitted to the intensive care unit after she became extremely short of breath 5 days after a hip replacement operation. What does it show?

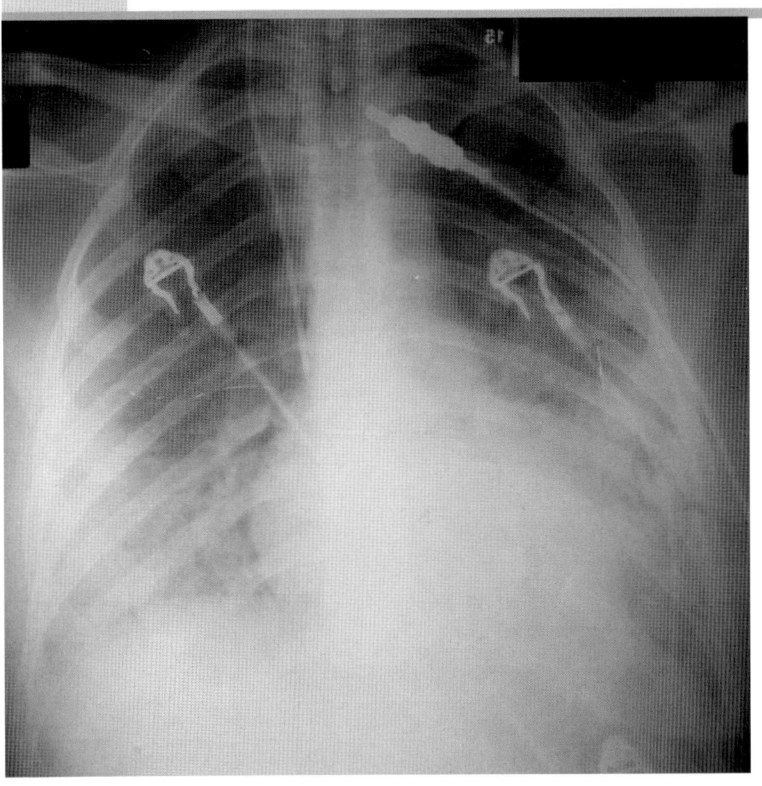

Initial impression

Bilateral white lungs.

Interpretation

This patient is obviously unwell. She has ECG leads and a right jugular line in situ. She also has bilateral white shadowing in the lower and mid zones of the lung. This could be bilateral pleural effusions, pulmonary oedema or consolidation. The whiteness is not homogeneous and if you look carefully, you can see the black outlines of the bronchi, especially in the right mid zone. This is what is meant by the term 'air bronchogram' and is a sign of consolidation. This woman had a severe, bilateral pneumonia.

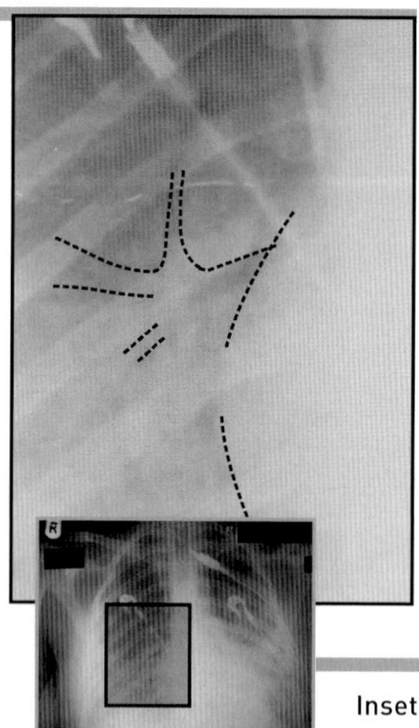

Inset: Branching dark structures known as air bronchograms.

SUMMARY

Severe hospital acquired pneumonia.

CXR 42

What abnormality is present on this lateral film?

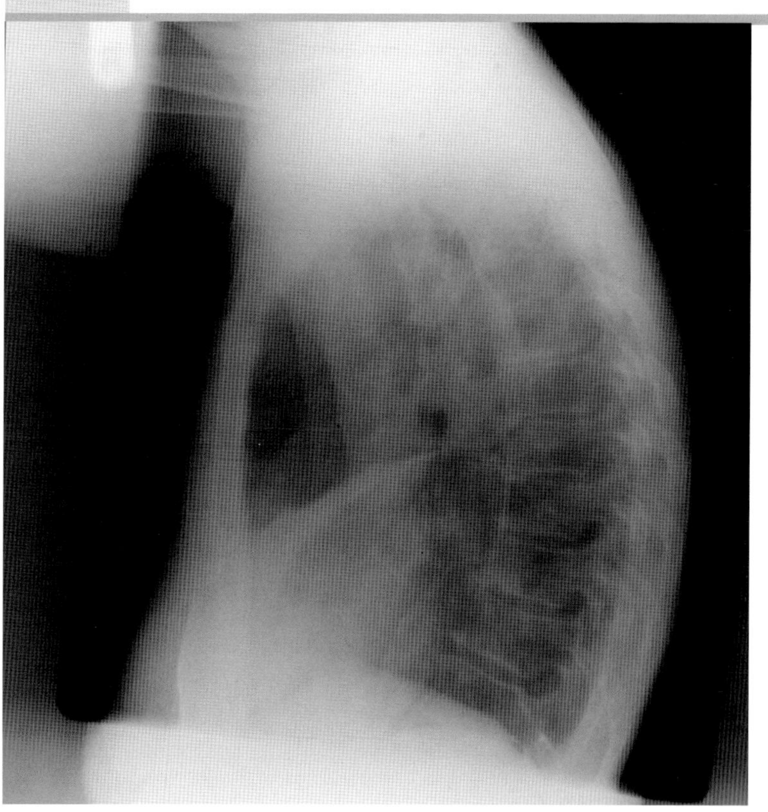

Initial impression

White shadowing.

Interpretation

There is an area of whiteness. Look carefully at the shape and borders of this whiteness. It is a triangle. The apex of the triangle is at the hilum and its base runs from the sternum to the diaphragm. This is the typical appearance of right middle lobe collapse. In fact this is lateral film taken of the patient described in CXR 36.

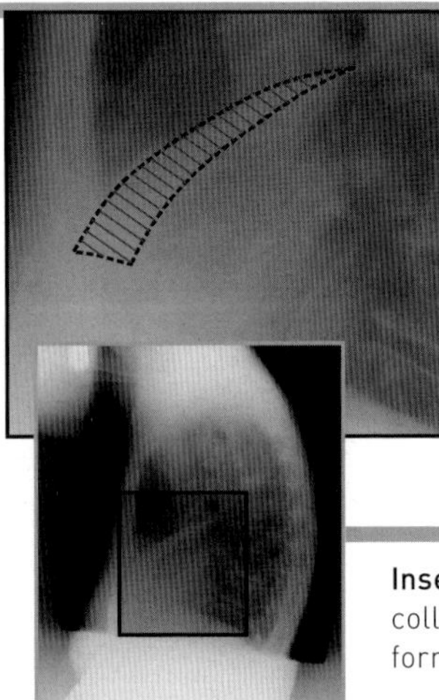

Inset: Typical appearance of a right middle lobe collapse on a lateral film. The upper margin is formed by the horizontal fissure.

SUMMARY

Right middle lobe collapse.

CXR 43

This 25-year-old man with a chronic productive cough attends as an out-patient once a year for a follow-up film. What is the underlying diagnosis?

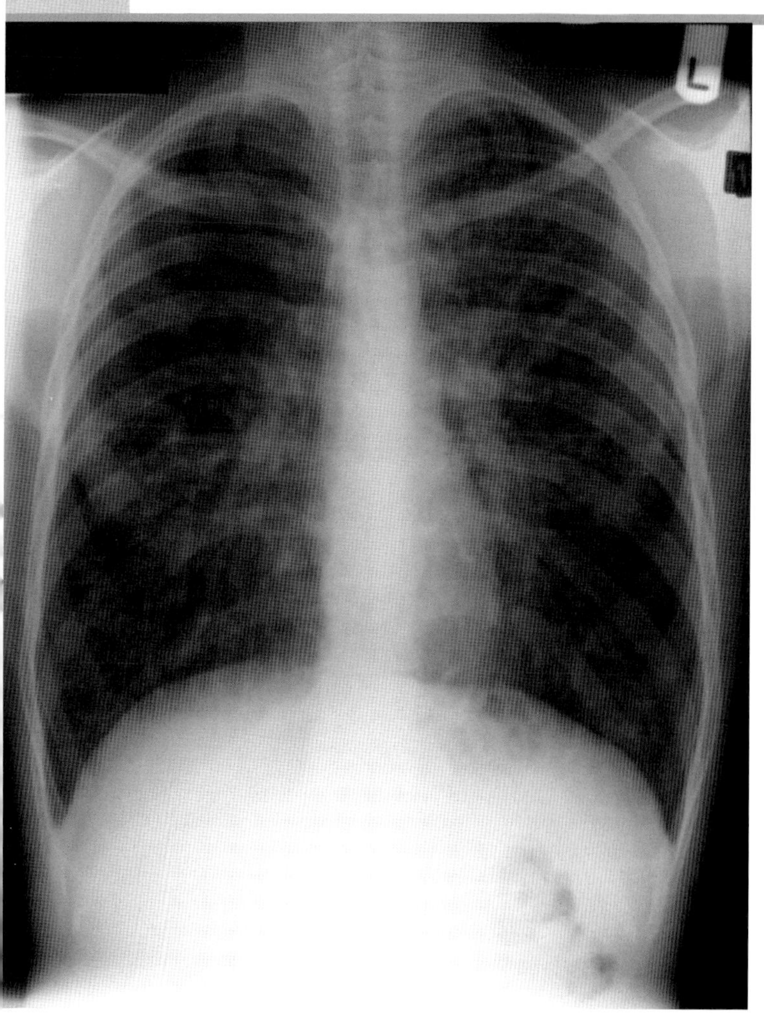

Initial impression

White lungs.

Interpretation

The film shows hyper-inflated lungs with eight anterior ribs visible above the diaphragm. There is very little subcutaneous fat around the lower chest so he has a low body mass index, which would fit with a chronic condition. There are white shadows in the lung fields, which predominate in the mid zones. Closer examination of these shows them to be ring-shaped shadows. These are caused by thickening of the bronchial walls and peribronchial inflammation. This is the typical appearance of bronchiectasis.

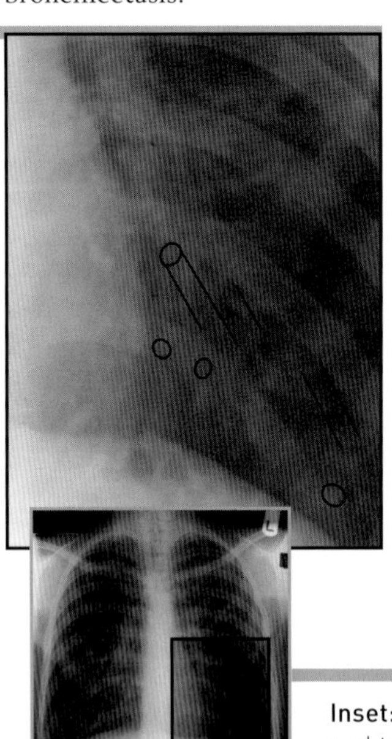

This patient has bronchiectasis which we know to be chronic since he has a low body mass index and hyper-inflated lungs. This young patient has cystic fibrosis.

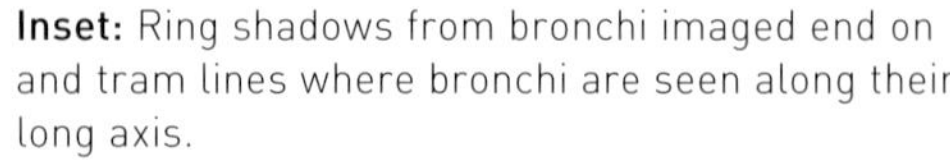

Inset: Ring shadows from bronchi imaged end on and tram lines where bronchi are seen along their long axis.

SUMMARY

Cystic fibrosis.

CXR 44

This 82-year-old woman was seen in the healthcare of the elderly clinic complaining of lethargy, marked weight loss and loss of appetite. What does her film show?

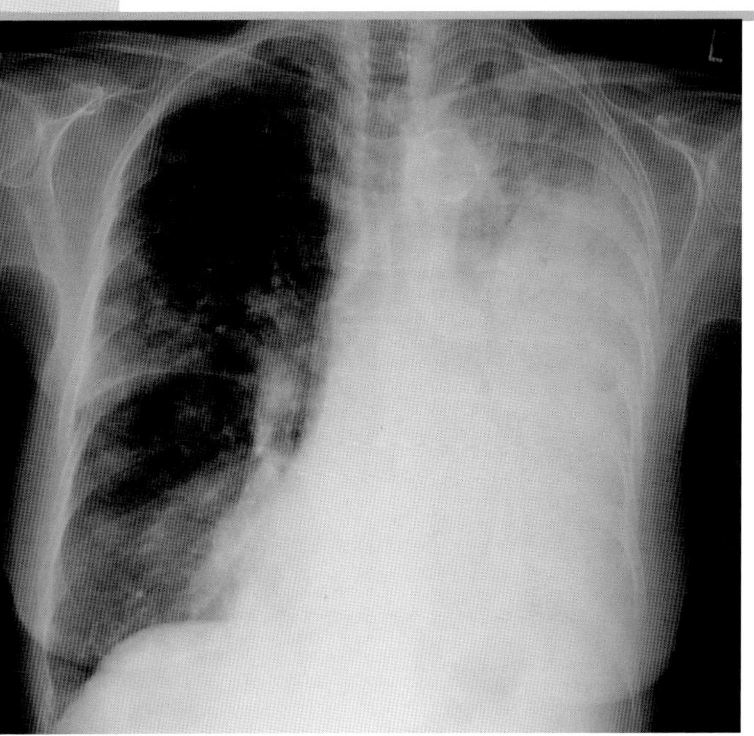

Initial impression

Extensive white lung on the left.

Interpretation

There is extensive white shadowing in the left lung. The bronchial tree can be clearly seen outlined in black against the white background. This is an air bronchogram due to patent airways against a background of consolidated lung. The commonest cause of this is infection but other things that will consolidate the air spaces, such as fluid, blood or malignancy, can all cause this appearance. In this case, the appearance was due to an adenocarcinoma and the patchy white changes on the right lung are due to the adenocarcinoma having spread to this area. The pathological diagnosis here is not important, but it is important that you are able to identify the air bronchogram.

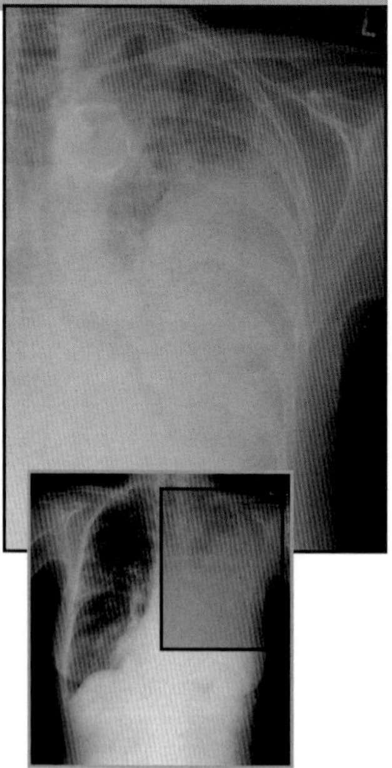

SUMMARY

Consolidation with air bronchograms.

CXR 45

This is a film of a 77-year-old man who presented to his GP with a history of haemoptysis and weight loss. Nothing was found on examination. Describe the film findings.

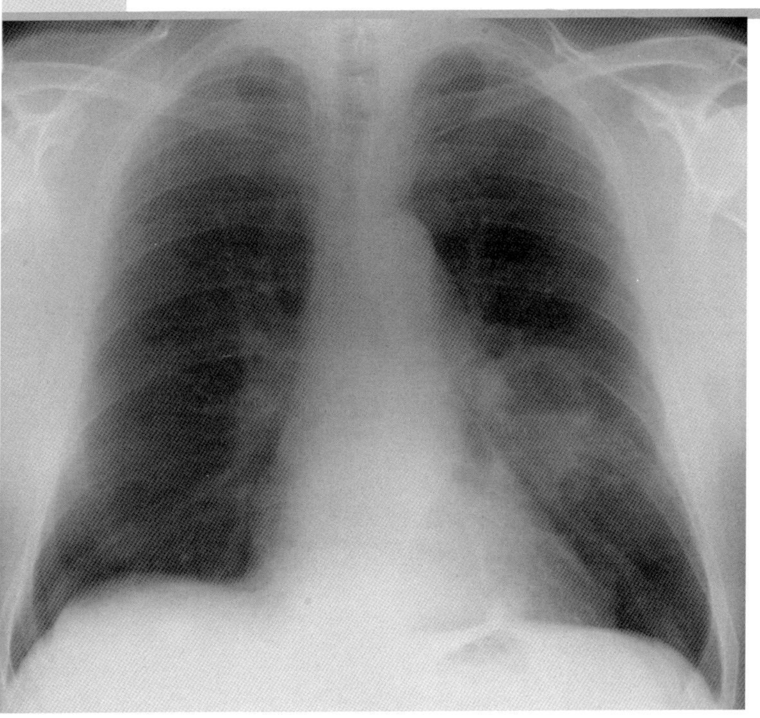

Initial impression

Large white shadow adjacent to the left hilum.

Interpretation

The shadow to the left of the hilum is a thick-walled cavity with an air/fluid level. An air/fluid level has a horizontal upper border with the fluid below being white and the gas above black.

A cavitating mass could be a malignancy or an abscess. To differentiate between the two, look carefully at the wall of the cavity. A wall with a thickness greater than 5 mm is more likely to be malignant. Always remember to look for other features of malignancy, for example bone metastases. There are none in this film.

This patient went on to have lung biopsy which confirmed a squamous cell bronchial carcinoma. Cavitating malignancies of the lung are usually primary bronchial carcinomas (in particular, squamous cell carcinomas), but occasionally metastatic tumours can cavitate.

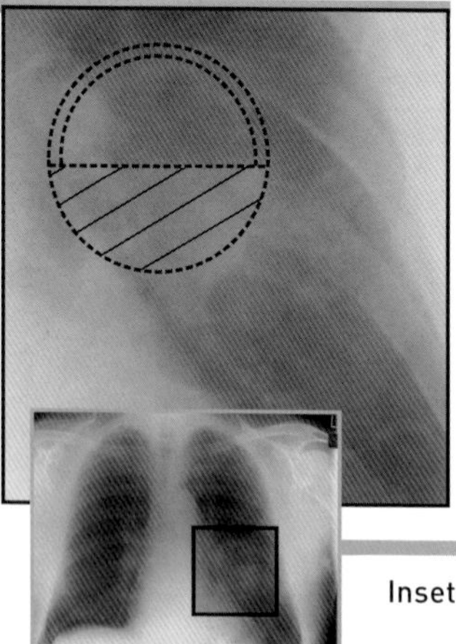

Inset: Air/fluid level in thick-walled cavity.

SUMMARY

Thick-walled cavity with air/fluid level.

CXR 46

(This is a follow-on film of the patient in CXR 19.) At bronchoscopy a blood clot was removed from the right main bronchus. This film was taken 2 hours after the bronchoscopy. What does it show?

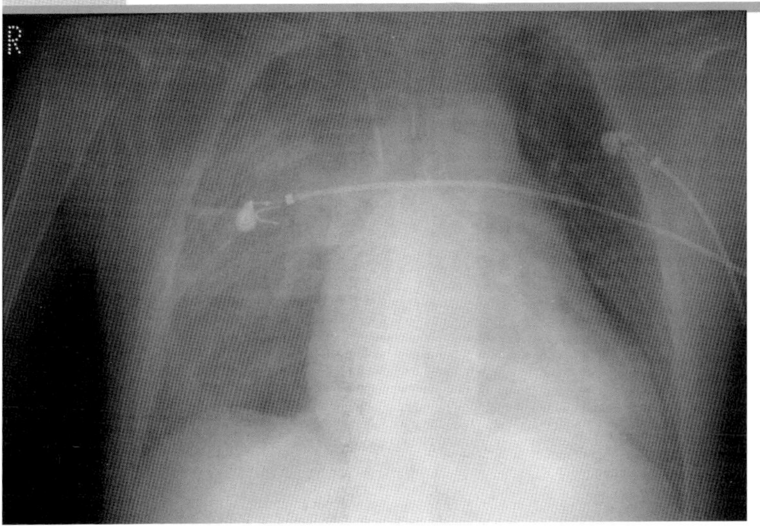

Initial impression

White right lung.

Interpretation

The patient is obviously in intensive care since an endotracheal tube and an internal jugular line are both visible. Also note that there is a second endotracheal tube within the left main bronchus. This was placed to protect the left lung, should the right lung re-bleed. There is still white shadowing on the right lung but the right bronchial tree is now patent and there is no mediastinal shift. There is residual whiteness that is patchy in nature and is due to residual blood within the air spaces.

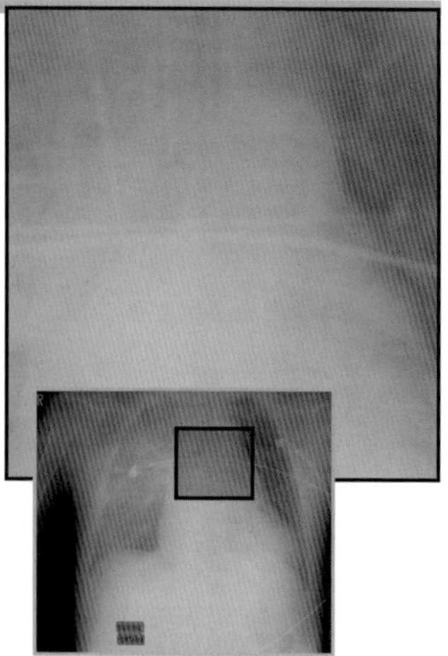

SUMMARY

Endotracheal intubation, with resolution of mediastinal shift and some consolidation.

CXR 47

This 81-year-old woman presented to the medical admissions unit with sudden onset of chest pain. How would you report this film?

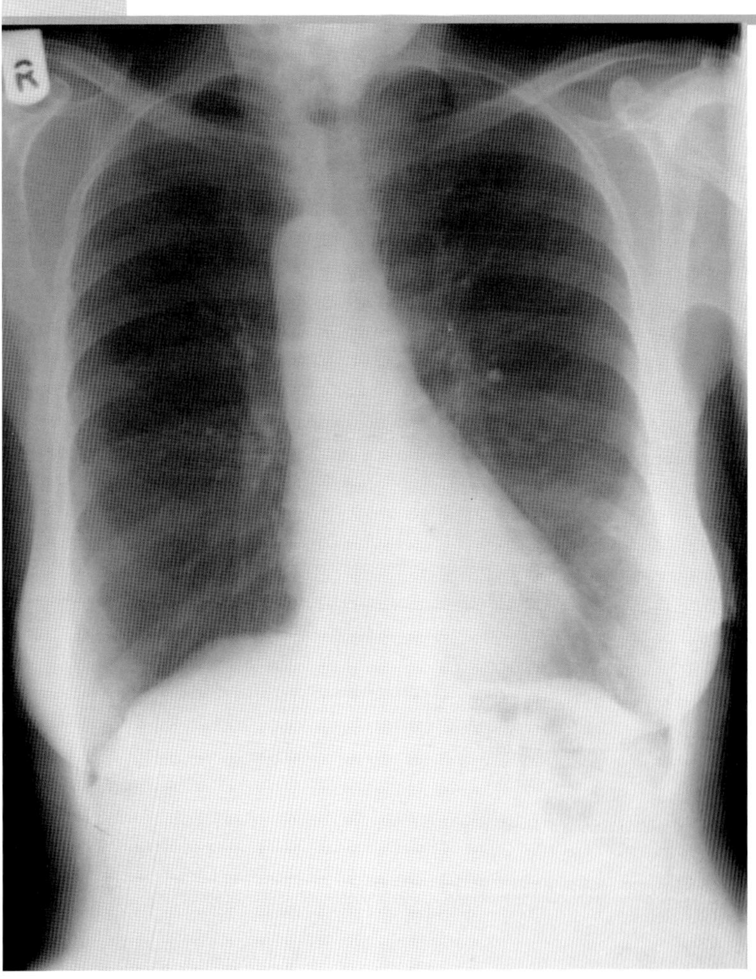

Initial impression

Abnormal mediastinum.

Interpretation

The lungs are clear and the heart size is normal. There is a vertical linear opacity to the right of the midline over the mediastinum. The upper border of this is curved and appears to contain some calcium. No left aortic arch is seen. The appearances are those of a right aortic arch, which in someone of this age is an incidental finding. This may be associated with abnormal origins of vessels from the aortic arch, which could form a ring around the trachea, producing airway problems. In an asymptomatic adult it would not warrant further investigation.

This right-sided aortic arch is an incidental finding and is not related to her chest pain.

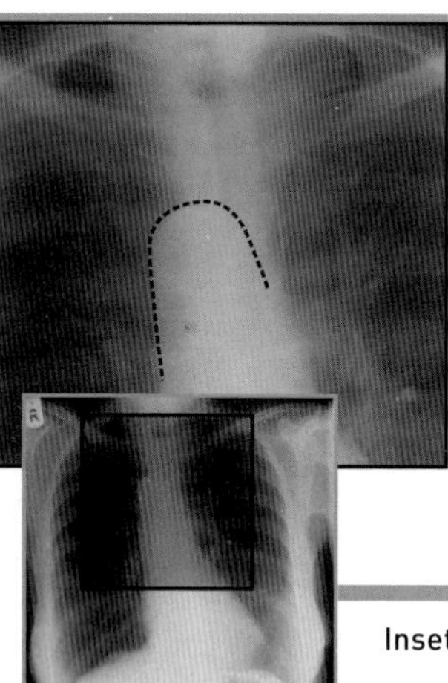

Inset: Right-sided aortic arch.

SUMMARY

Right-sided aortic arch. No cause for chest pain is identified.

CXR 48

This 68-year-old woman developed increasing shortness of breath over a period of 2 weeks. She was a heavy smoker but was otherwise fit and well. What would be your major concern with this woman?

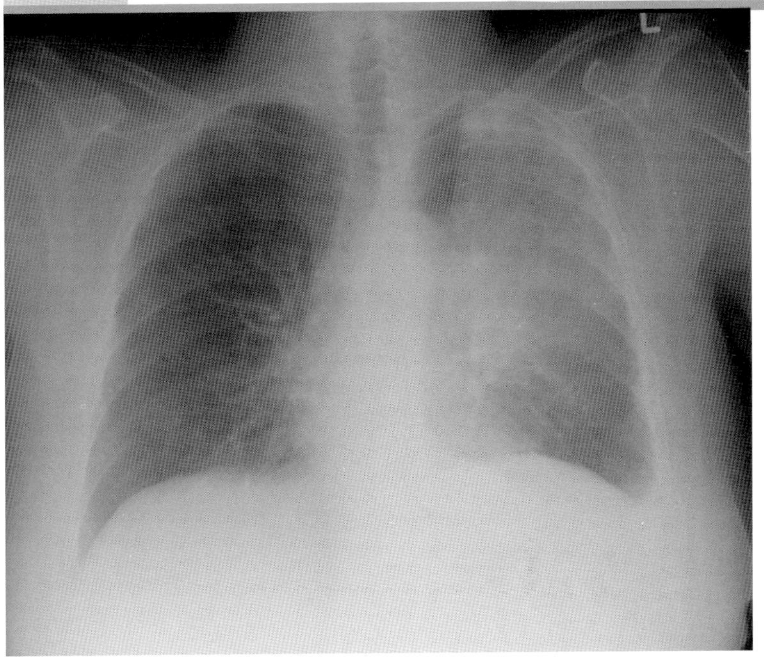

Initial impression

White left lung.

Interpretation

The left lung field is white compared to the right. This could be due to consolidation, a pleural effusion or lung collapse. An effusion is unlikely since the whiteness is not homogeneous, is not basal in distribution and does not obscure the diaphragm. No air bronchogram is visible, making consolidation less likely.

This film shows left upper lobe collapse, which is often described as looking like a veil over the left lung field. The area is not totally white, as the lower lobe lies behind the upper lobe, not below it. The crisp contours around the aortic knuckle and left pulmonary artery are usually lost. Other features that are sometimes visible on a PA film include tracheal and maybe cardiac shift to the left, and elevation of the left hemidiaphragm.

The collapse of the left upper lobe anteriorly can be seen in a lateral view, with a band of whiteness at the front of the chest, making the retrosternal window whiter than normal.

The major concern in this heavy smoker would be that the left upper lobe collapse was due to a central bronchial carcinoma. A CT scan and a bronchoscopy demonstrated a tumour obstructing the left upper lobe bronchus.

SUMMARY

Left upper lobe collapse from carcinoma.

CXR 49

This is the film of a 50-year-old man who presented to the emergency department with severe abdominal pain. What does the film show?

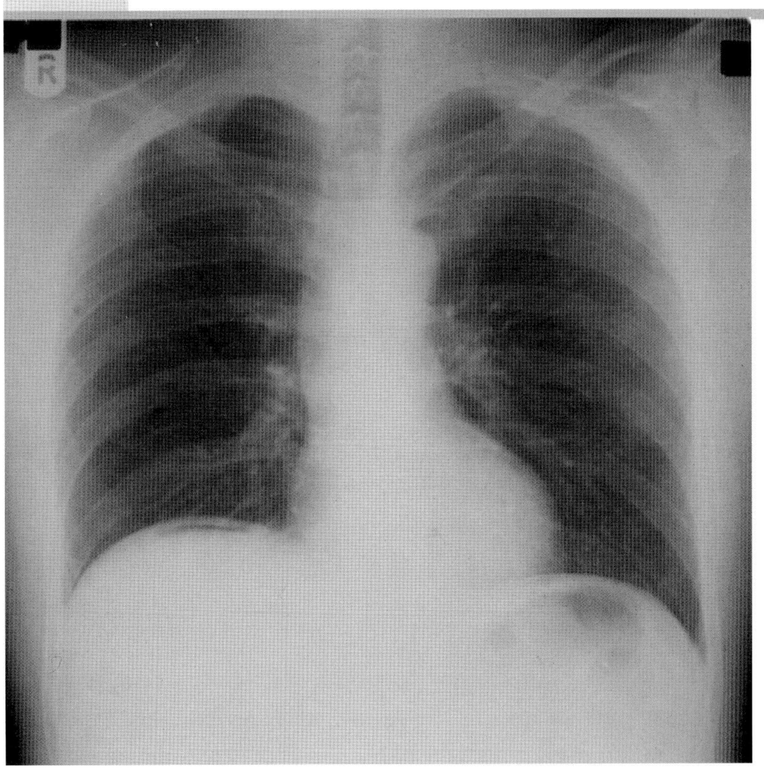

Initial impression

Abnormal area under the diaphragm.

Interpretation

When looking at a film, always remember to do a full survey. In this case the abnormality is under the diaphragm where there is a rim of black. In the context of the clinical history, this could be free air under the diaphragm, but it could also be an area of gas within the gut, interposed between the liver and the diaphragm – a normal variant, known as Chilaiditi's syndrome.

It can be difficult to distinguish Chilaiditi's syndrome from free air under the diaphragm. Look carefully at the area of blackness for signs of bowel markings. In this film, no bowel markings are visible within the area of blackness and the blackness is due to free air under the diaphragm.

Sometimes further investigations are needed to determine whether air under the diaphragm is free or within the gut. A simple method is to lay the patient on their left side for around 10 min, and take a film of the right lateral chest at the level of the diaphragm. Free air will move around to lie between the liver and the chest wall, unlike gas retained by bowel that will remain in the same position.

This man had free air under the diaphragm due to perforation of the bowel.

SUMMARY

Free air under the diaphragm.

CXR 50

This 59-year-old man was sent by his GP for a chest film as he was complaining of some pleuritic left-sided chest pain. Why did the radiologist suggest repeating the film?

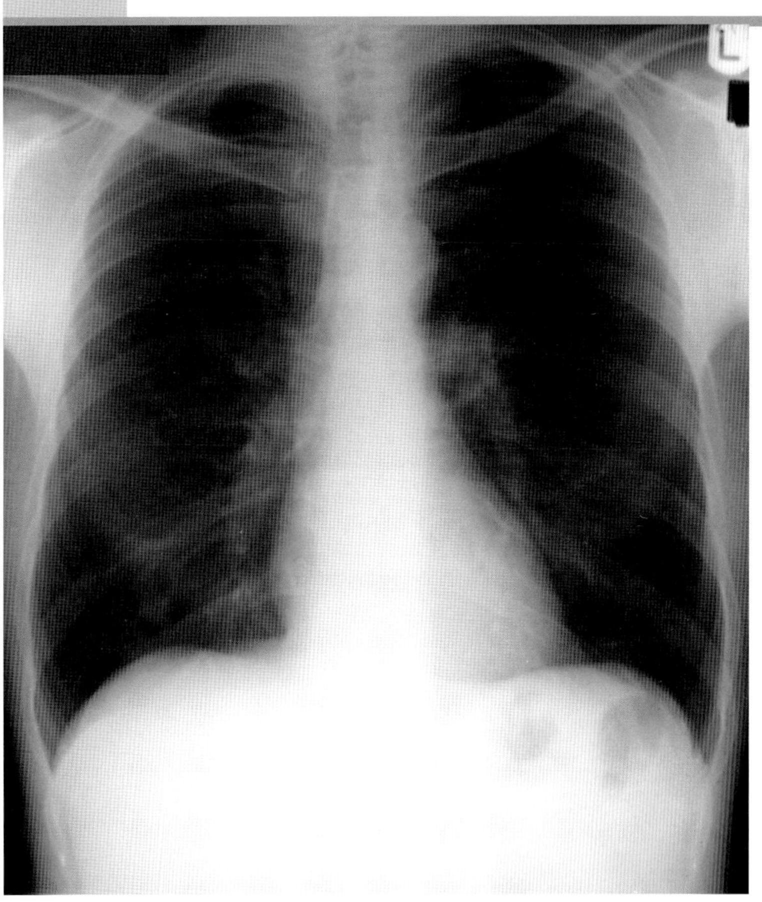

Initial impression

No obvious abnormality.

Interpretation

Bearing in mind the history given and the age group that this patient falls into, a pneumothorax, focal chest infection or a rib lesion should be considered. The presence of a pleural reaction should also be looked for.

Look at the right lower zone of this film and you will see a small 1.5 cm opacity. It appears to be positioned (projected) between the 6th and 7th anterior ribs in the mid-clavicular line. If there is an opacity like this on each side, it is highly likely that the appearance will be due to nipple shadows. A unilateral opacity, however, could be a lung nodule. An easy way to sort this out is to perform another film with a marker over the nipple.

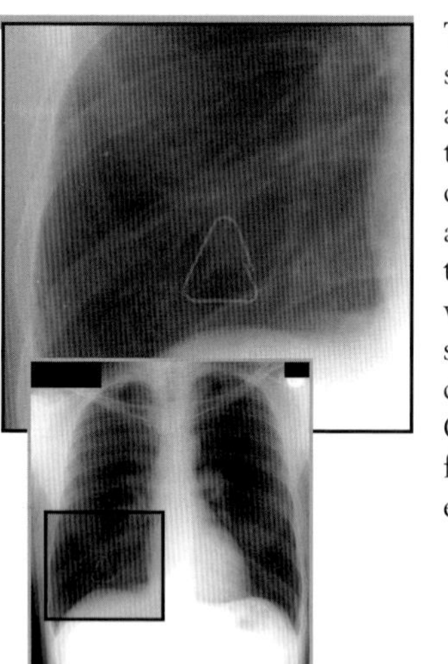

The follow-up film shows a marker surrounding the lung lesion, confirming it as a nipple shadow. Nipple shadows tend to be oval. They have a well-defined circumference but usually there is an area where the margin is blurred. This is the portion of the nipple in continuity with the chest. Some patients have other skin tags on the chest, which can cause confusion, and to prevent an unnecessary CT scan of the chest, the skin on the front and back of the chest should be examined.

SUMMARY

Nipple shadow. The radiologist suggested repeating the film with nipple markers.

CXR 51

This 75-year-old woman presented with abdominal and chest pain, and shock. What is the diagnosis?

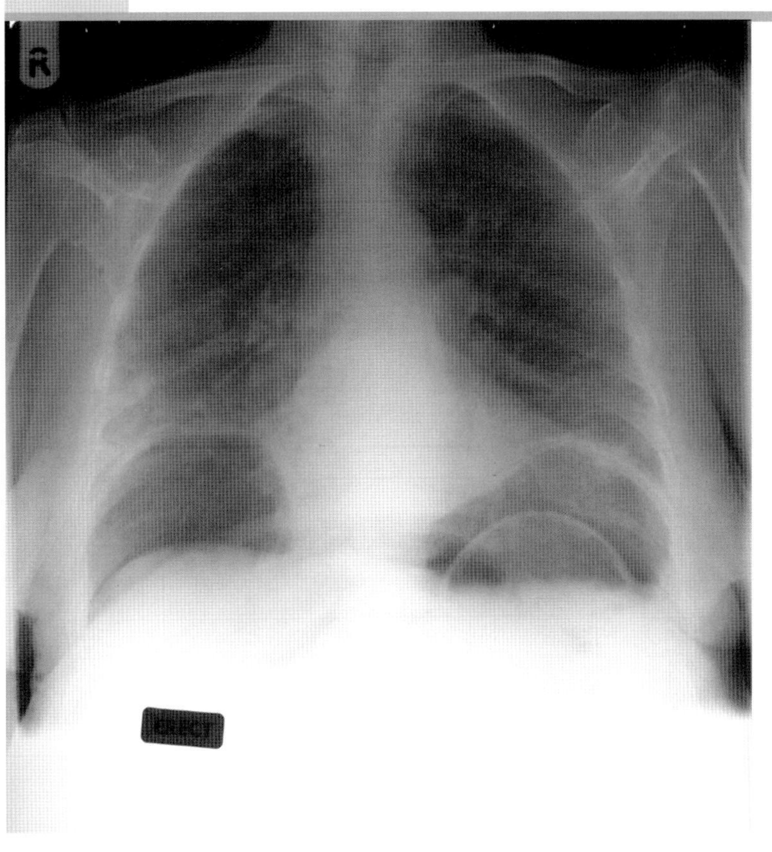

Initial impression

Abnormal blackness at the bottom of both lungs.

Interpretation

The diaphragmatic contours on both sides are abnormally high. Look at the area under the diaphragms. This area should be opaque due to the presence of the abdominal organs, but in this film the area appears black. The black appearance is due to air or gas under the diaphragm, in this case due to perforation of the bowel. Under the left hemidiaphragm a loop of bowel can also be seen – probably colon. Look how clearly the outer wall of the bowel appears. This is because there is air both within and outside the bowel allowing both the inner and outer wall of the bowel to be visualized. Usually only the inner border of the bowel wall is visible. This abnormal appearance is called Rigler's sign and indicates perforation of a hollow viscus – usually due either to peptic ulceration of the stomach or duodenum, or a colonic perforation.

The heart appears diamond shaped. This is because there is an area of atelectasis (small areas of collapsed lung) next to the heart. The atelectasis has occurred because the raised diaphragm has pushed on the lung, causing small areas of collapse.

SUMMARY

Extensive bilateral free subphrenic gas due to gut perforation, leading to peritonitis, and sepsis.

CXR 52

This 65-year-old woman visited the gastroenterology clinic, with a recurring history of swallowing problems. This film was taken. What does it demonstrate?

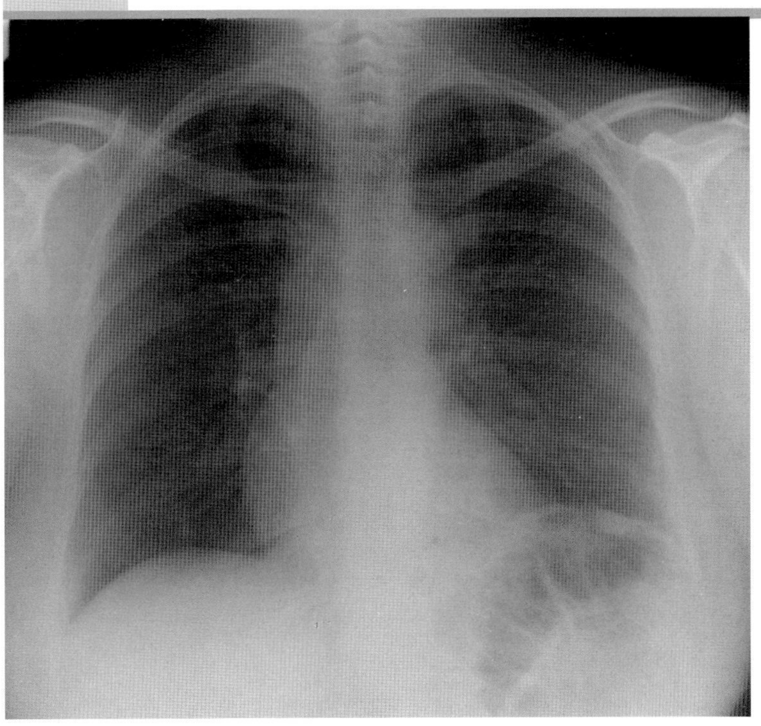

Initial impression

A difficult film, which on first inspection may look normal.

Interpretation

Before dismissing a film as normal it is important to look at areas where subtle abnormalities can be missed. You need to look at the lung apices, the heart shadow, the area behind the heart, the mediastinum, as well as the area below the diaphragms. Look also for subtle hilar abnormalities. The clinical history and examination findings should help you focus on areas where any abnormalities are likely to occur.

This woman has swallowing problems so look carefully at the mediastinum and the area behind the heart. To the right side of the mediastinum is a white line curving outwards. It does not fit anatomically with an area of lung, as it crosses the boundaries of the upper and lower lobes. The linear appearance is because it is a structure outlined by gas – air in the lung laterally, and gas within the oesophagus centrally. The line is the wall of the oesophagus and the oesophagus is visible here because it is dilated. This may be due to achalasia (abnormal oesophageal motility) or a distal stricture, which could be malignant. The recurrence of symptoms would suggest that this is a benign lesion, and treatment may be oesophageal dilatation for a stricture.

SUMMARY

Dilated oesophagus.

CXR 53

This is a lateral film from Case 29, where it was not possible to determine whether the consolidation was in the left upper or lower lobe. Has the lateral helped?

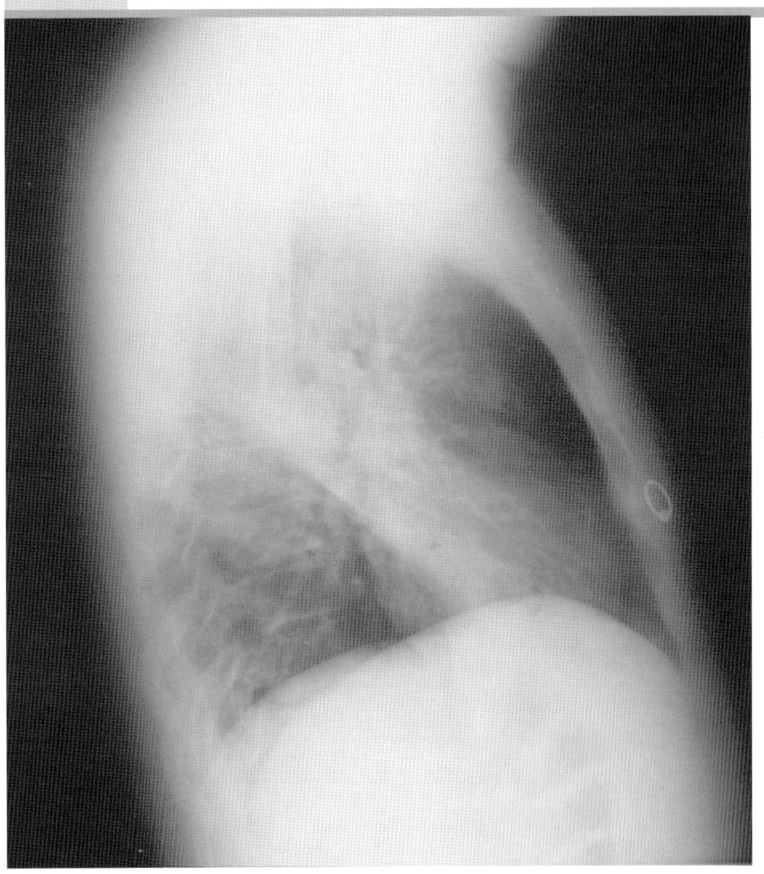

Initial impression

The consolidation lies in the middle of the film.

Interpretation

The retrosternal window is dark so it is normal. The oblique fissure is more clearly seen than normal and this is because the consolidation lies adjacent to the fissure, lying just in front. This indicates that the consolidation in the left mid zone lies within the upper lobe. The lower lobe is clear. The lateral view of the thoracic spine quite clearly shows the thoracic spine, becoming more clearly defined, and the image darker going down the vertebral column, which is normal.

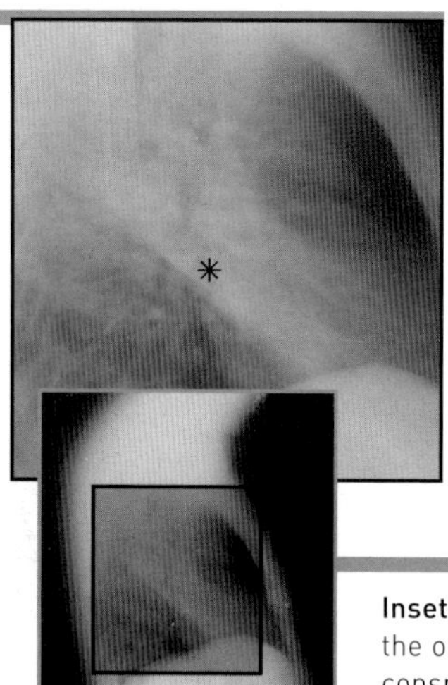

Inset: Consolidation lies in the upper lobe against the oblique fissure,* making it much more conspicuous.

SUMMARY

Area of consolidation confirmed as being in the left upper lobe.

CXR 54

This 84-year-old woman was admitted to the emergency department with sudden onset of severe shortness of breath. This is the portable film taken on admission. What does it show?

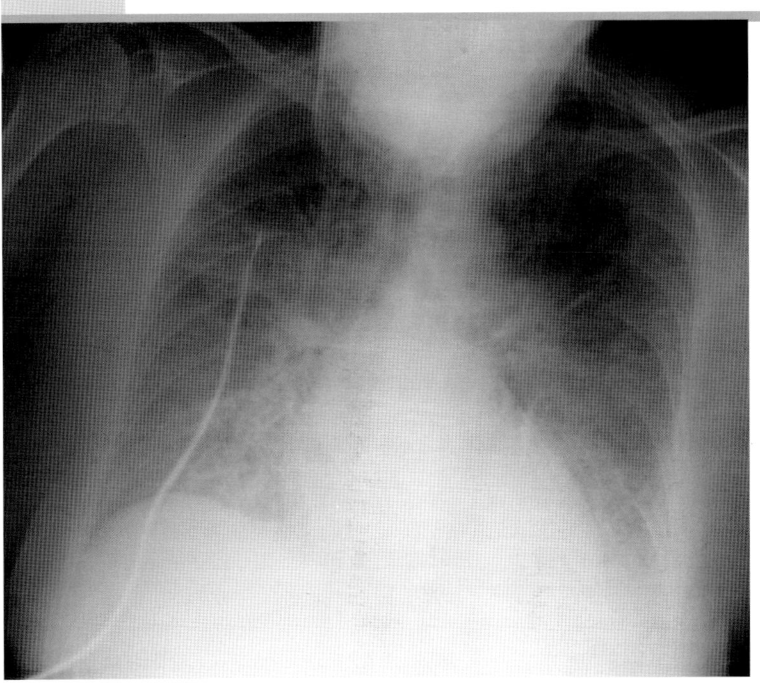

Initial impression

Technically imperfect film in a sick woman showing increased whiteness in the lung fields.

Interpretation

Initial survey of this film shows a number of features that suggest the patient is unwell. It is an AP film and the patient is clearly wearing an oxygen mask. It has obviously been difficult to position the patient properly since she is not central on the film and her head and oxygen mask obscure the top of the chest suggesting she was unable to keep her head raised.

Closer examination of the lung fields shows diffuse whiteness of the lungs in the lower zones and around the hilum. This is not homogeneous shadowing but has an alveolar type appearance. Superimposed on the shadowing are numerous straight lines radiating from the hilum, and additional horizontal lines abutting the chest wall, so-called Kerley B lines. Both of these lines are caused by venous congestion and fluid in the lymphatics. The perihilar nature of the shadowing and the presence of interstitial lines indicate that this patient has pulmonary oedema, the most likely cause of which is left ventricular failure. The left hemidiaphragm is not clearly seen and in this area the white shadowing is more homogeneous in nature. This is a small left pleural effusion secondary to the pulmonary oedema. No comment can be made on the heart size since this is an AP film. As is often the case in very sick patients the difficulty in obtaining a technically adequate film means that it is not possible to make out any upper lobe blood diversion.

Most pleural effusions associated with heart failure are bilateral or right sided. In this case the effusion is left sided because the patient has been lying on their left-hand side.

SUMMARY

Acute pulmonary oedema.

CXR 55

This well 34-year-old nurse had this film taken as part of her application for a Canadian visa. What is the abnormality shown?

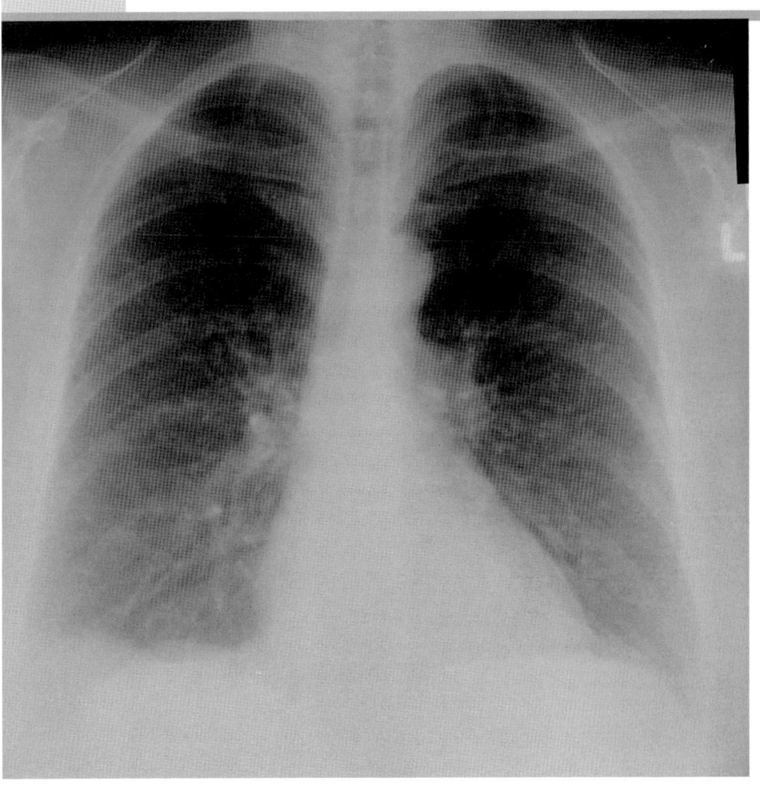

Initial impression

White, nodular shadowing.

Interpretation

There are numerous small nodules throughout both lung fields. The differential diagnosis would include previous chicken pox pneumonia, tuberculosis and multiple miliary metastases. To distinguish between these you need to look at the number, distribution and type of nodules. The distribution is in the lower and mid zone which is typical for old chicken pox pneumonia. There are a limited number of nodules, probably less than 100, which would go against tuberculosis. Close inspection of the nodules shows them all to be a similar size and density. Their dense nature is due to calcification, which would exclude miliary tuberculosis. Some lung metastases can calcify, but this is almost always after chemotherapy, and the clinical history excludes this. The calcification,

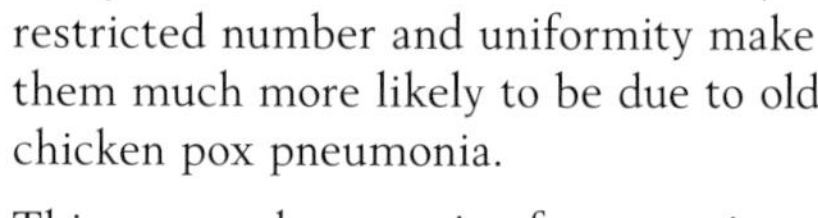
restricted number and uniformity make them much more likely to be due to old chicken pox pneumonia.

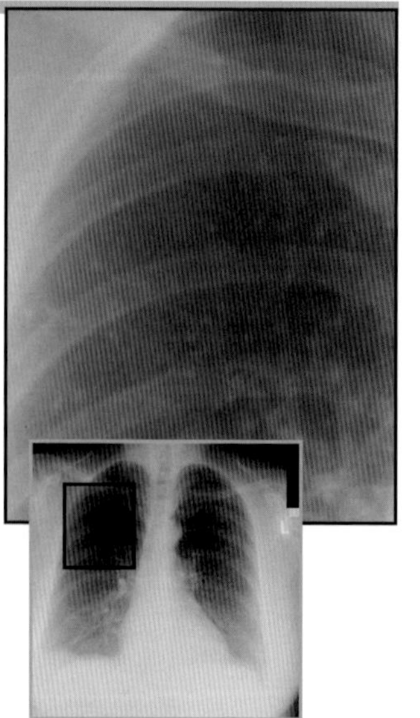

This woman has scarring from previous chicken pox pneumonia.

SUMMARY

Previous chicken pox pneumonia.

CXR 56

This 55-year-old man was admitted following a 2-week history of increasing shortness of breath, and swinging fevers. On admission he was found to have a large right pleural effusion, and a chest drain was inserted. This confirmed the presence of an empyema. What complication has occurred?

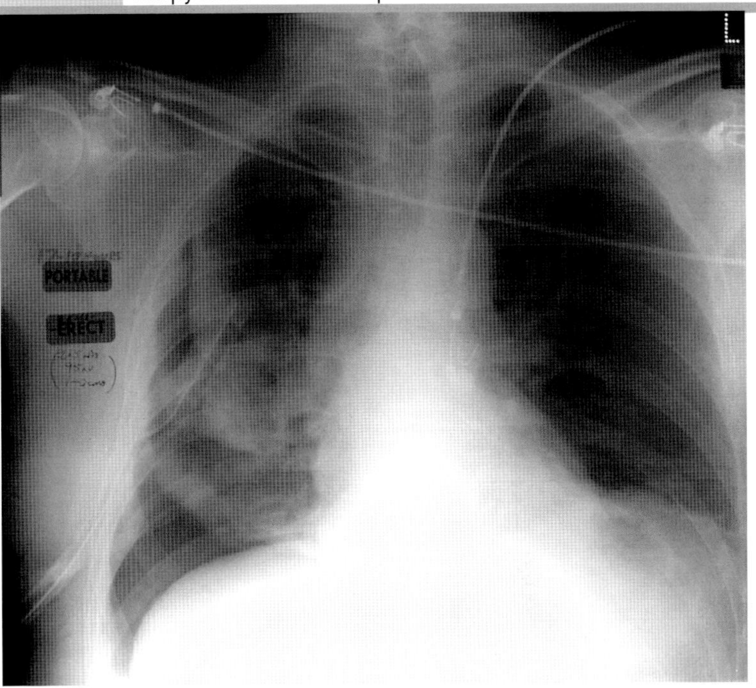

Initial impression

Abnormal white and blackness in the right chest. There is a chest drain in situ.

Interpretation

There is a right-sided chest drain and ECG leads are present. This is an AP erect film.

There is a pneumothorax on the right, lying mainly underneath the collapsed portions of the right lung, but a small amount of air can also be seen around the apex. In most cases of pneumothorax, the lung and pleural margin is a thin white line only 1–2 mm across. In this case, however, there is a much thicker rind of soft tissue around the lung on the right and it extends into the fissures. This is known as trapped lung because the lung is no longer being compressed by the effusion but it cannot re-inflate either as the visceral pleura has thickened and encased it. This appearance can occur with either infection or malignancy, especially a mesothelioma.

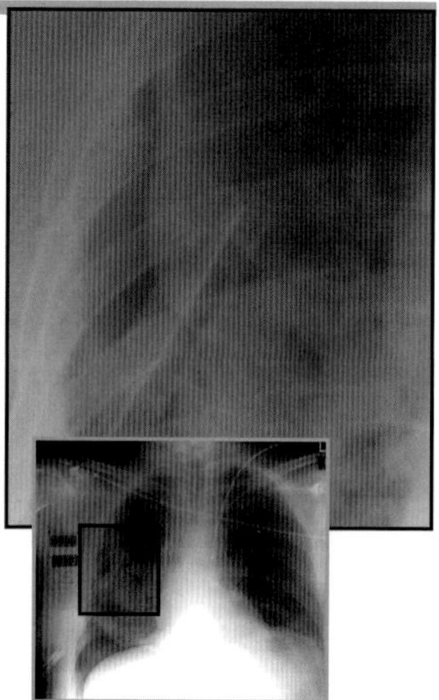

SUMMARY

Trapped lung from visceral pleural thickening.

CXR 57

This 63-year-old man presented with a 4-month history of increasing shortness of breath and lethargy. Clinical examination revealed an early diastolic murmur and a pansystolic murmur suggestive of aortic regurgitation and mitral valve disease. What radiological features support this diagnosis? Why is the patient short of breath?

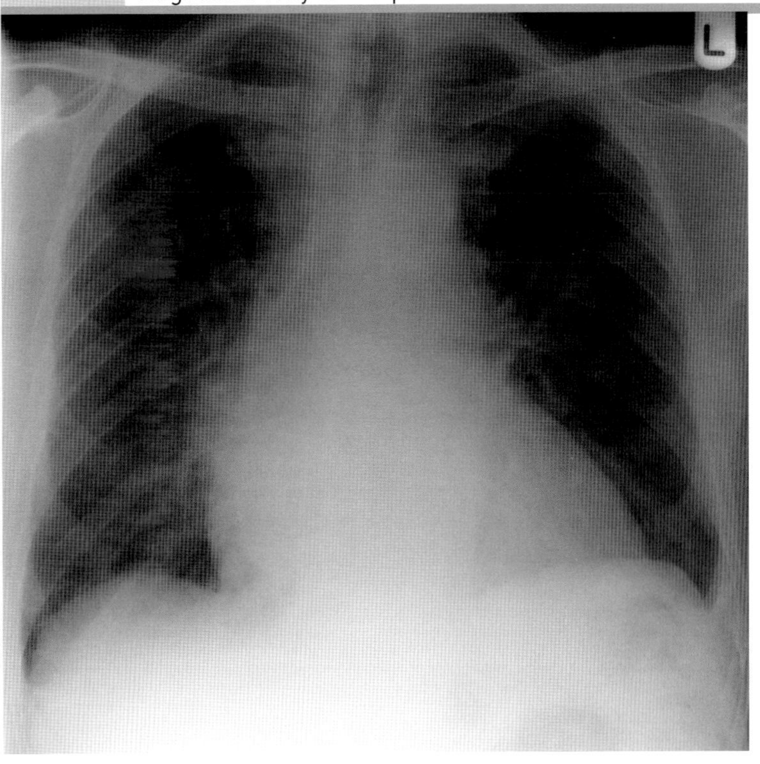

Initial impression

Abnormally shaped heart in a patient with valvular heart disease.

Interpretation

Always remember to look at the heart when you examine the chest X-ray. The first thing to notice is that the heart is enlarged since it is more than half the size of the thoracic diameter. After observing cardiac enlargement, you should look very carefully at the shape of the heart – the cardiac outline. Observe the right side of the heart shadow. In this X-ray you can see a double heart border which is a feature of left atrial enlargement. This occurs because the left atrium is situated behind the heart and when it is enlarged it can be seen through the right atrium. Note also the splaying of the carina – the angle between the two main bronchi should be less than 90°. This is caused by the enlarged left atrium pushing the left main bronchus upwards. This appearance can also be due to a mass in the subcarinal region.

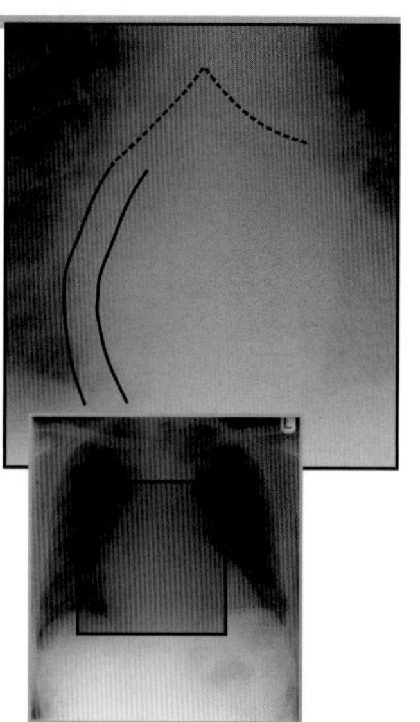

In the lung fields you can see Kerley B lines – horizontal non-branching white lines, which are up to 2 cm in length. These are a sign of pulmonary oedema, a common complication of mitral valve disease. This would explain the patient's breathlessness.

SUMMARY

Double right heart border and splaying of the carina due to an enlarged left atrium. This patient has pulmonary oedema secondary to mitral and aortic valve disease.

CXR 58

This 30-year-old man was feeling generally unwell. A blood test showed him to be hypercalcaemic. What does the film show?

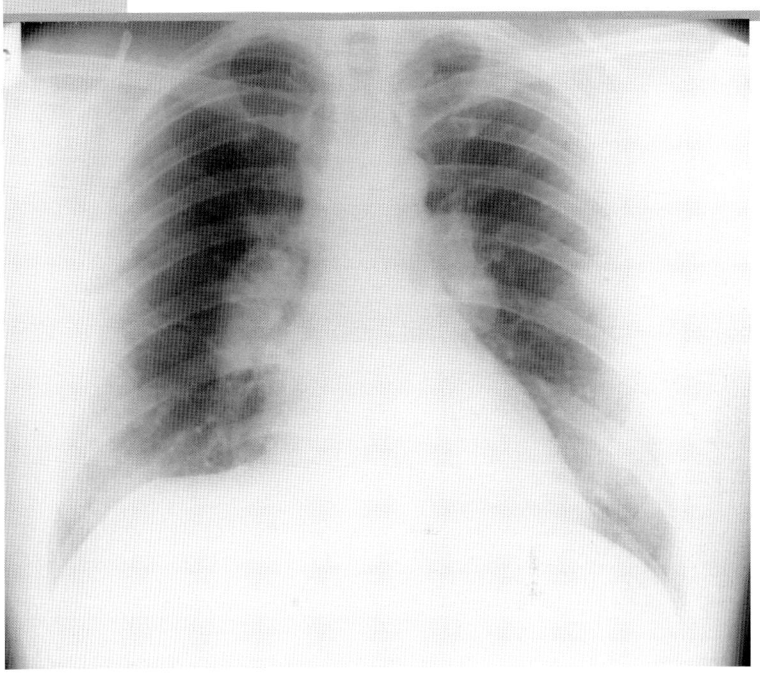

Initial impression

Abnormal hila.

Interpretation

At first glance the film looks very abnormal, with a lot of whiteness around the edges. The whiteness extends out peripherally beyond the lungs and chest wall, and represents extensive subcutaneous fat. This makes the film difficult to interpret.

Allowing for the obesity, the lung fields themselves look normal, but the hila appear large, the right side more so than the left. Assessing the size of the hila is a matter of experience. If you are uncertain, compare this film to one that you know is normal. In this film, not only do the hila appear large but the normal concave shape is lost. This is another sign of hilar enlargement.

This patient has bilateral hilar lymphadenopathy. With this clinical history the most likely cause is sarcoidosis.

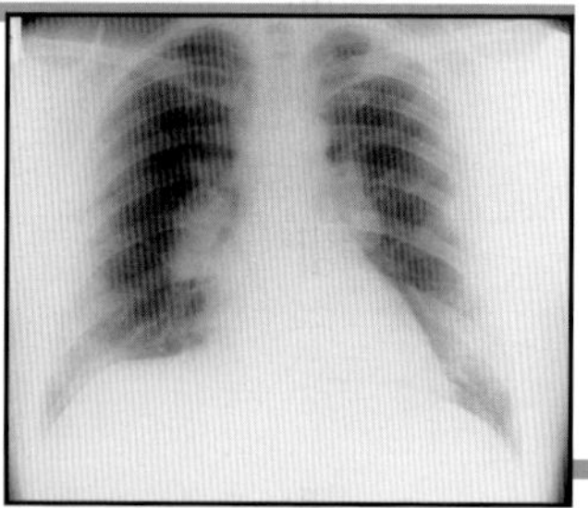

Above: Obesity causes increased whiteness along the lateral chest wall. In a woman with large breasts, increased density can be seen over the lower zones and bases.

SUMMARY

Bilateral hilar lymphadenopathy.

CXR 59

What are the abnormalities on this film of a 62-year-old woman?

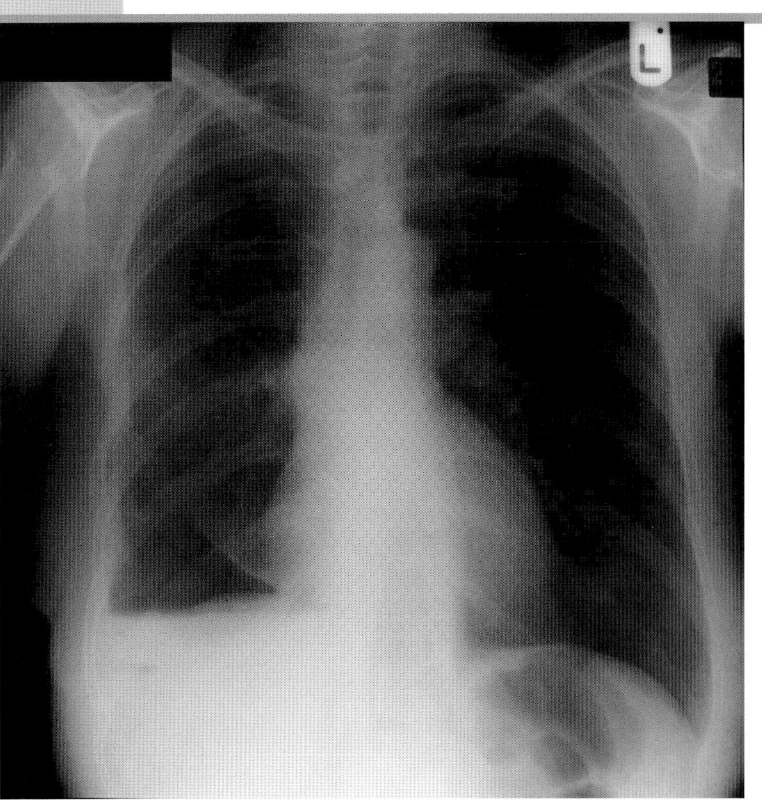

Initial impression

Whiteness of the right lung base.

Interpretation

There is an area of abnormal whiteness at the right lung base. This could be due to consolidation or a pleural effusion. The homogeneous nature of the whiteness goes against consolidation. There is no obvious meniscus, which you would expect with a simple pleural effusion. Instead, the upper border is straight, which occurs with an air/fluid level. This is the typical appearance of a hydropneumothorax, i.e. a pleural effusion with air above it.

Do not stop there! A full survey of this film gives other information. The right 6th rib is missing, the right hilum is smaller and lower than you would expect and there are curved white lines in the right lower zone, above the hydropneumothorax. The right 6th rib was removed because this patient had a right lower lobectomy and this appearance may occur following such a procedure. Eventually the space that was left when the lung was removed will be taken up by the diaphragm moving up and the mediastinum shifting to the right. This has not yet happened and so, on this film, the space is filled with fluid and air.

SUMMARY

Right lower lobectomy with hydropneumothorax.

CXR 60

This 43-year-old man, known to be infected with human immunodeficiency virus, presented with fevers, a dry cough and feeling generally unwell. What diagnosis is suggested by the film?

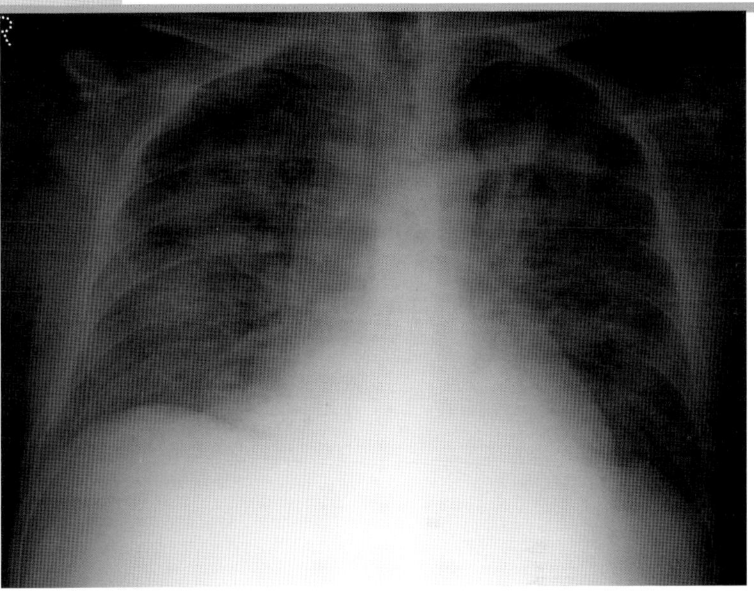

Initial impression

Both lungs abnormally white.

Interpretation

The shadowing is around both the left and right hilum more marked the right than left. Look carefully at the nature of this shadowing. It is vague and the underlying blood vessels and airways can still be seen. This is the so-called 'ground glass' appearance. There are numerous causes of ground glass shadowing but in this patient *Pneumocystis carinii* pneumonia would be the most likely cause.

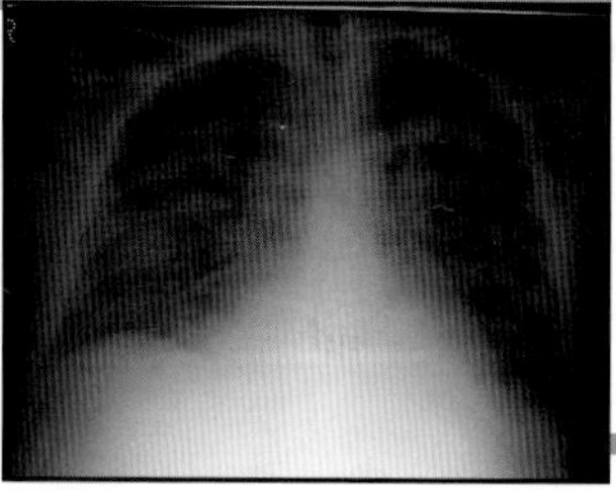

Above: Diffuse hazy shadowing making the vessels in the lung more difficult to identify.

SUMMARY

Pneumocystis carinii pneumonia.

CXR 61

This 32-year-old woman has a congenital vascular abnormality. The pulses in her arms are good, but the femoral arterial pulses are weak, and there is radiofemoral delay. She presents with headaches and high blood pressure. What diagnosis does the film suggest?

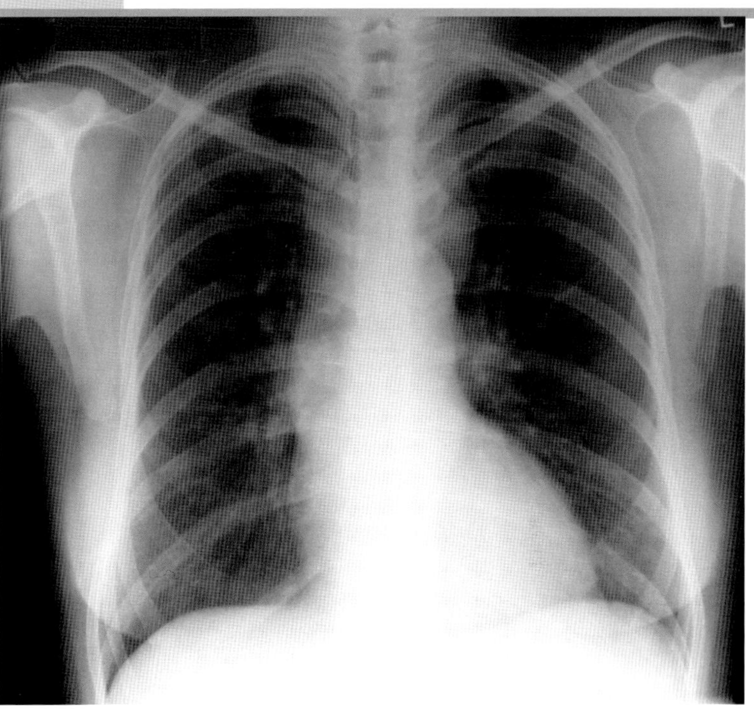

Initial impression

Abnormal whiteness of the upper portion of the mediastinum.

Interpretation

The clinical history of a vascular abnormality and the increased whiteness in the superior mediastinum suggests this could be the aorta. A fall in blood pressure between the arms and legs suggests aortic narrowing. The suggestion here is that this is aortic coarctation. The coarctation is most commonly found on the distal arch just beyond the origin of the left subclavian artery. As the blood from the aorta needs to by-pass the stenosis, collateral vessels enlarge. The posterior fourth to seventh ribs demonstrate notching of their inferior borders. This is due to enlargement of the intercostal arteries. The first 3 ribs are not generally involved. In this case the aortic arch has become aneurysmal, leading to the superior mediastinal density. The heart size is normal.

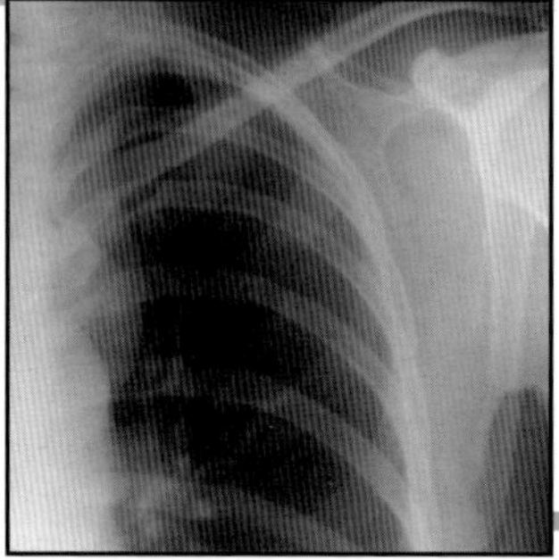

Above: Enlargement of the intercostal arteries causes notching of the inferior borders of posterior ribs.

SUMMARY

Aortic coarctation with rib notching, and an aneurysmal aortic arch.

CXR 62

This 82-year-old retired civil servant presented with a 6-week history of a dry cough. His GP referred him to the lung clinic after receiving a worrying report on this film. How would you interpret the film and what further investigation would you do?

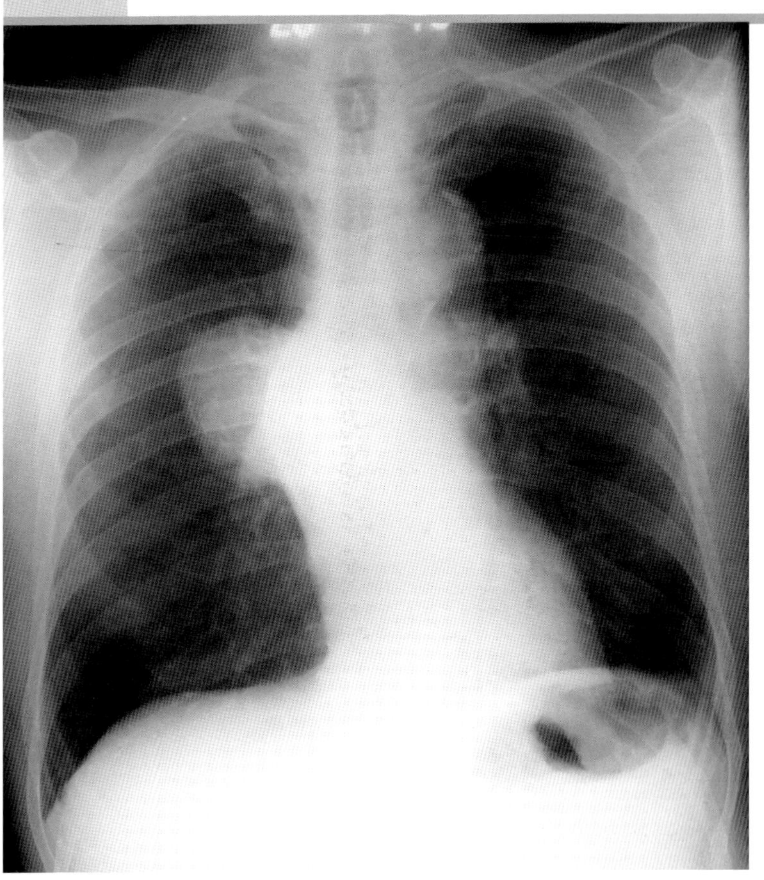

Initial impression

Abnormal right hilum.

Interpretation

There is an abnormal density over the right hilar area and it has a smooth rounded convex appearance. A normal sized pulmonary artery can be seen through the density. Increased density in the hilar area may be due to abnormally large lymph nodes, enlarged blood vessels, or to masses behind or in front of a hilum. It is often difficult to distinguish these. This is a particularly difficult film. The smooth edge suggests a vascular structure, as opposed to either lymphadenopathy which would be more lobulated, or a mass which might have a more spiculated appearance. The contours of the ascending aorta can also be identified, which goes against an aortic aneurysm.

To define this further, CT scanning is necessary. In this case, the scan revealed the mass to be a saccular aneurysm. coming from the ascending aorta. The aneurysm has a narrow neck, so most of the contour of the ascending aorta is preserved which is why it can be clearly seen in this film.

This is not the typical appearance of an aortic aneurysm. We have included it to stress how difficult it can be to make this diagnosis from a plain film alone.

SUMMARY

Saccular ascending aortic aneurysm.

CXR 63

Why is this 45-year-old civil servant short of breath?

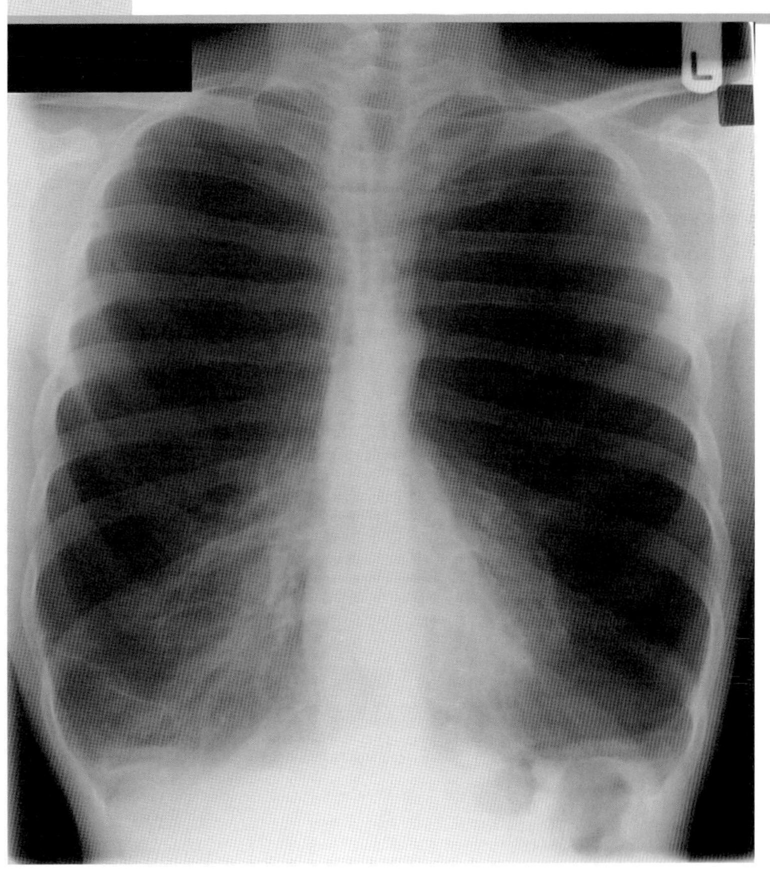

Initial impression

Bilateral black lungs.

Interpretation

Both lung fields look black. Black lungs could be due to over-penetration of the film, pneumothoraces or bullous lung disease. You need to decide which of these it is.

This film does not appear particularly over-penetrated. Bilateral pneumothoraces would be rare (though not impossible) and no lung edge is visible, which you would expect to see with a pneumothorax.

This film demonstrates a number of features of hyperinflated lungs, which would suggest chronic obstructive pulmonary disease as the most likely diagnosis. The diaphragms are flattened and pushed down and the heart appears to be thin and 'floating' above the diaphragm. Look at the ribs – they appear more horizontal than usual. Count the number of ribs visible anteriorly – there should only be seven ribs visible whereas in this case you can count nine.

The hyperinflation of the chest suggests chronic obstructive pulmonary disease. The blackness of the lungs is likely to be due to bullous emphysema. The unaffected lung has been squashed by the formation of bulla and now occupies a small area in the lower zones of this film. This appears denser than normal lung because it has been compressed by the emphysematous bullae.

This man has severe chronic obstructive pulmonary disease at a young age. It would be important to check his alpha-1 antitrypsin levels. In this case they were normal.

SUMMARY

Chronic obstructive pulmonary disease.

CXR 64

This 24-year-old IT operator reported to his GP with a cough and pleuritic chest pain. The GP ordered this film. Is any treatment necessary?

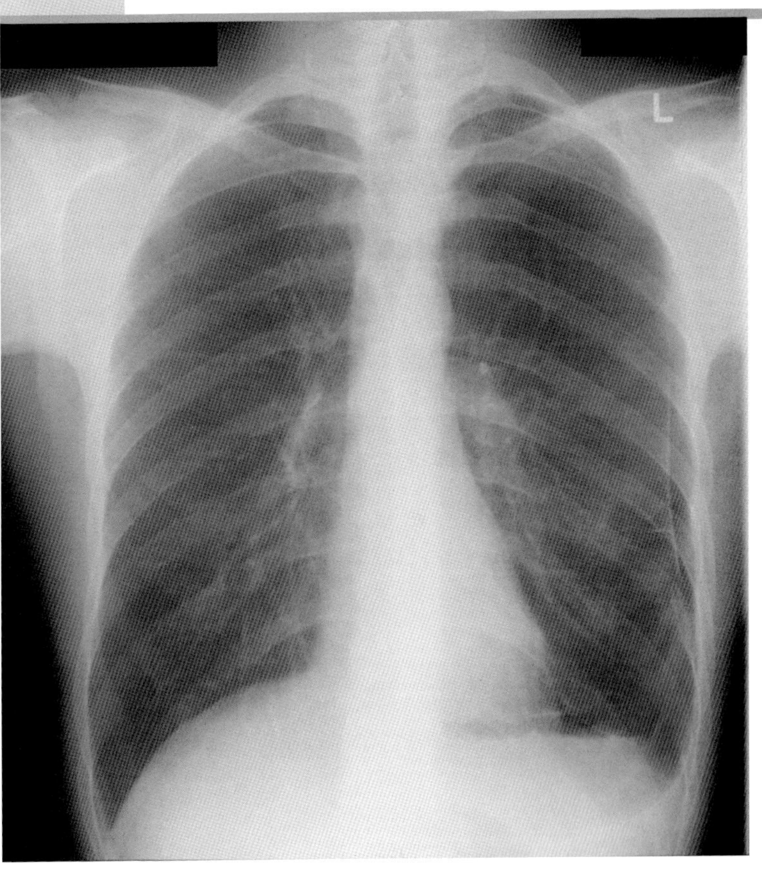

Initial impression

Area of black left lung.

Interpretation

Close inspection shows an area of blackness in the periphery of the left lung field. There are no lung markings visible in this area and the convex edge of the lung can be clearly seen. This is a pneumothorax.

In a 24-year-old otherwise fit man, this is most likely to be a primary pneumothorax. However, you do need to survey the rest of the lung field to check that there is no underlying lung disease. In this case the rest of the lungs look normal.

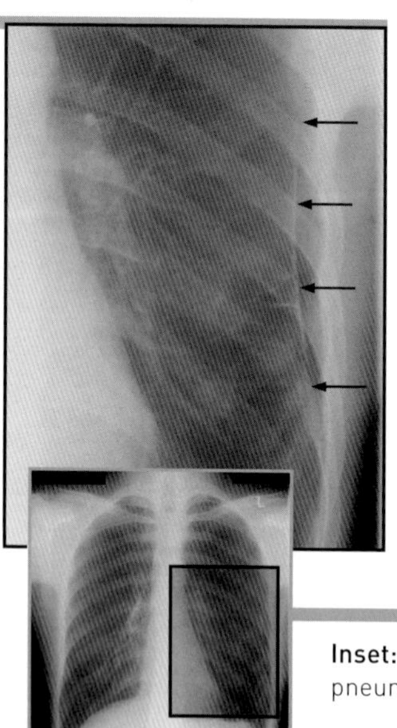

This is a primary pneumothorax that is less than 2 cm in size and is therefore considered to be small. The patient is not breathless so no treatment is necessary, unless it becomes a recurring problem.

Inset: The arrows show the edge of a small lateral pneumothorax.

SUMMARY

Small primary pneumothorax. No treatment is necessary.

CXR 65

This 84-year-old man presented with gradually increasing breathlessness. This was the film on admission. What is the most significant abnormality?

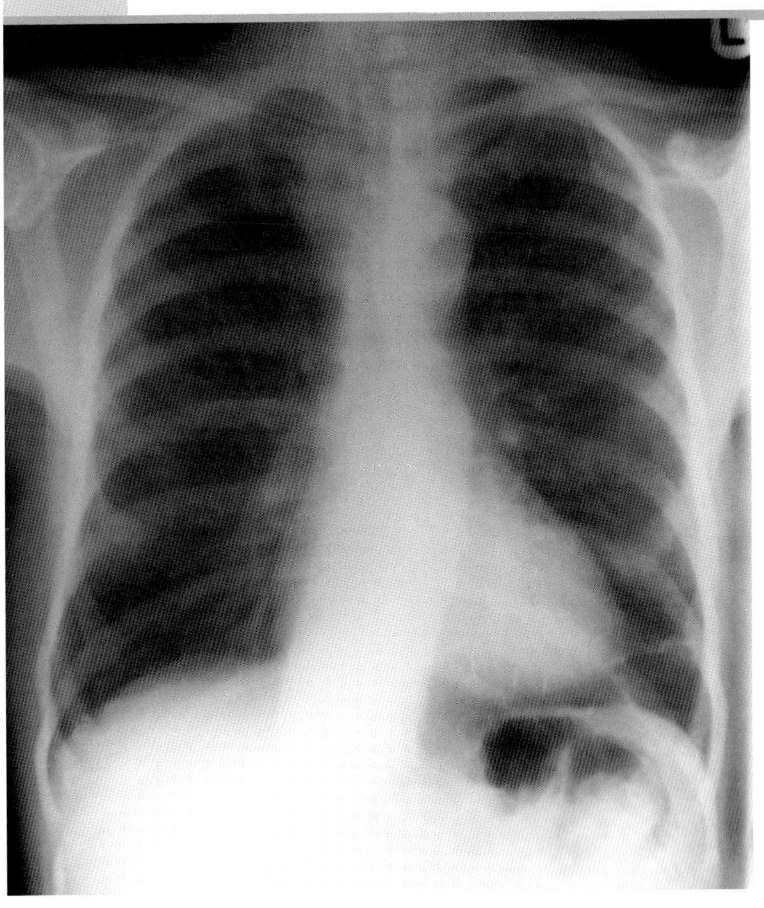

Initial impression

Lungs and mediastinum look normal.

Interpretation

We mention several times throughout this book the importance of review areas and here is another case. The heart and mediastinum appear normal, and other than a small linear scar at the left lung base, the lungs appear clear.

By now you will have checked the apices, behind the heart and under the diaphragms. Examine the bone texture. You will see that the bones look denser than normal. A normal rib will usually have a thin dense white margin and the central portion of the bone will appear less dense, as it is seen from the side. In this case, however, the ribs and clavicles appear diffusely white. This is because the patient has sclerotic bony metastases. In an elderly man the most likely cause will be advanced prostate cancer.

Potential causes for his breathlessness would include renal failure secondary to bladder outflow obstruction. Anaemia is possible, either from blood loss from the primary tumour, or with so many metastases he may not be able to form blood within his marrow properly.

SUMMARY

Sclerotic bony metastases.

CXR 66

This is the film of a 60-year-old man with a six-month history of breathlessness and a dry cough. What does the film show?

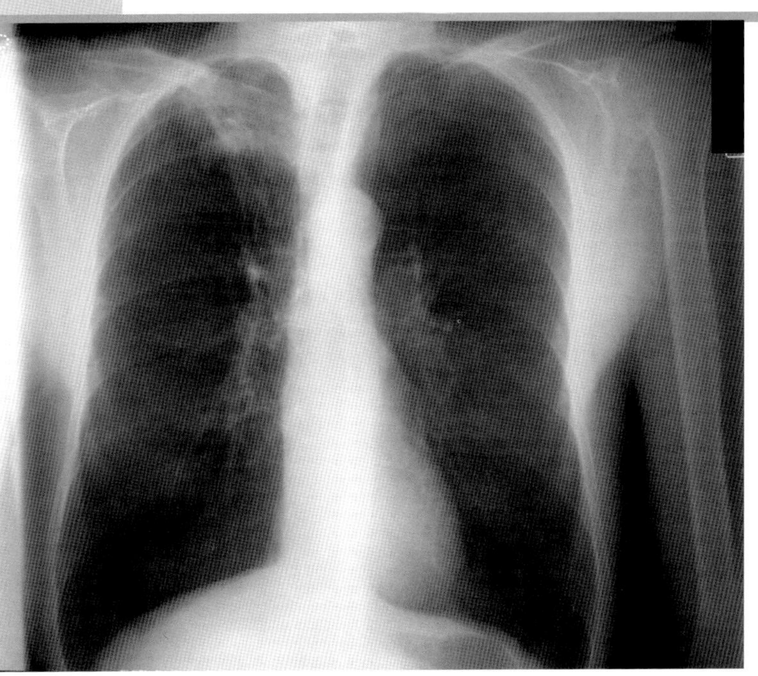

Initial impression

White lung.

Interpretation

There is white shadowing across both lung fields and the diaphragm and mediastinal borders have a shaggy appearance. Close inspection of the shadowing shows it to be mesh-like in appearance – this is termed reticular shadowing and is a typical appearance of fibrotic lung disease. Look at the distribution of the shadowing, which is more pronounced at the bases. This distribution of the shadowing and the clinical history is most suggestive of cryptogenic fibrosing alveolitis.

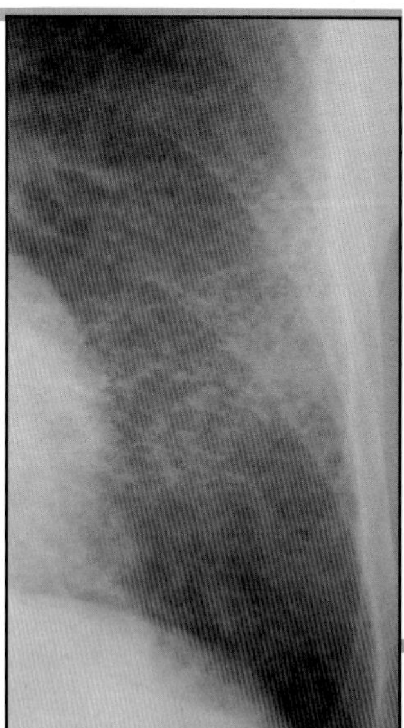

Left: Reticular shadowing at the left lung base.

SUMMARY

Cryptogenic fibrosing alveolitis.

CXR 67

This patient has recently had an operation. What has she had done and what complication has developed?

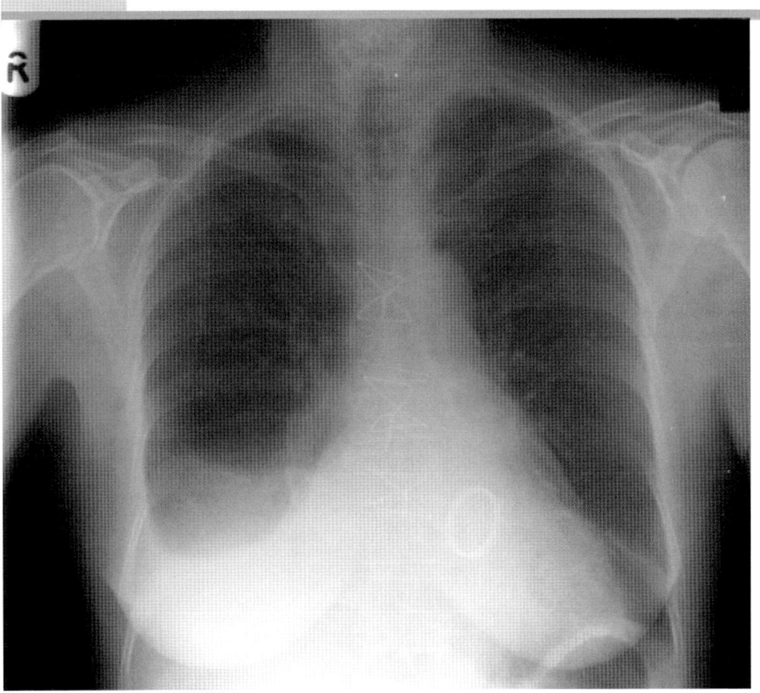

Initial impression

Abnormal white density in the right lower zone.

Interpretation

There are metallic wires tied in a figure of eight in the midline indicating a sternotomy. To the left of the midline is a rounded metallic density representing a metallic prosthetic heart valve. This woman has had a mitral valve replacement.

At the right lung base is an area of increased whiteness. Looking at the upper margin of this will help to determine the cause: the curved upper border being higher laterally than in the midline is in effect a form of meniscus indicating that the whiteness is due to a pleural effusion.

Within the lungs there is also a linear band at the left lung base close to the apex of the heart. This is a common post-surgical finding, and is due to poor respiratory effort, or some retained secretions causing a small area of collapse. Small areas of collapse such as this are called areas of atelectasis.

SUMMARY

Post-mitral valve replacement, with basal atelectasis and a right basal effusion.

CXR 68

This 35-year-old man complained of a chronic dry cough, lethargy and loss of appetite. He was referred to the chest clinic after his GP received the report on this film. Why is the film abnormal and what would be the differential diagnosis?

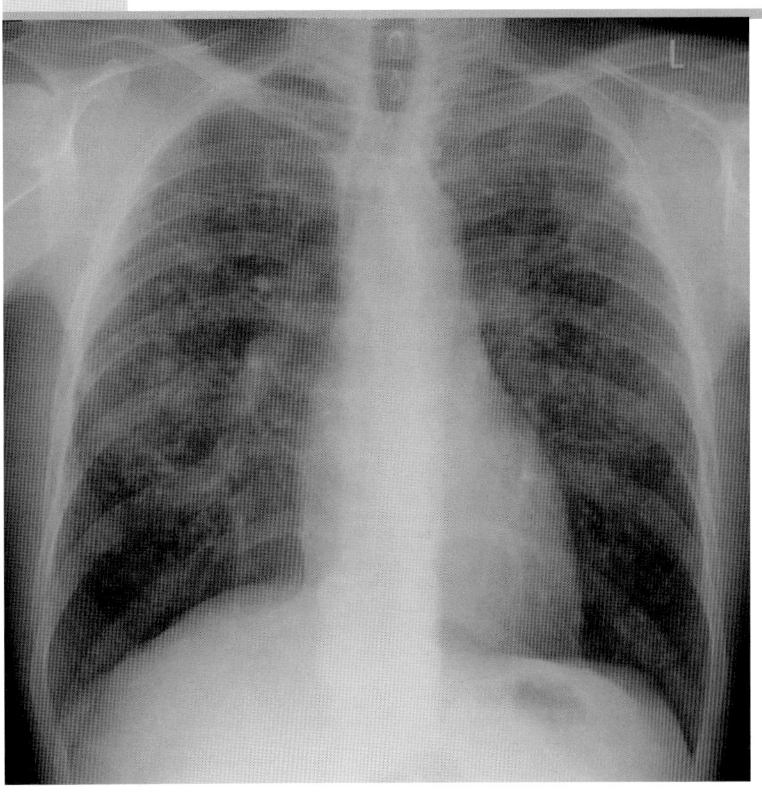

Initial impression

Bilateral abnormal white lung.

Interpretation

Both lungs appear whiter than they should and close inspection shows this to be due to multiple white nodules. The hila are obscured partially by these lung nodules but are not grossly enlarged. You need to characterize the distribution and nature of the nodules to determine their likely cause. Look first at their distribution. In this film they are most numerous in the mid and upper zones, a distribution most commonly seen with sarcoidosis. Other causes of this distribution would include pneumoconiosis, but this would not fit with the clinical history. Metastatic deposits tend to have a peripheral and basal distribution. Look also at the nature and number of the nodules. Chicken pox pneumonia scarring produces small, 3 mm, slightly irregular calcified nodules, usually less than 100 in number. Miliary tuberculosis causes multiple nodules of the same size in a widespread distribution. Post-primary tuberculosis in someone immunosuppressed might cause this appearance.

This patient had sarcoidosis and the differential diagnosis of this film would include post-primary tuberculosis, old chicken pox pneumonia, metastatic deposits or industrial lung disease.

SUMMARY

Sarcoidosis.

CXR 69

This 89-year-old woman was brought in to the medical admissions unit with a history of confusion. What can you tell about her previous medical history from this film?

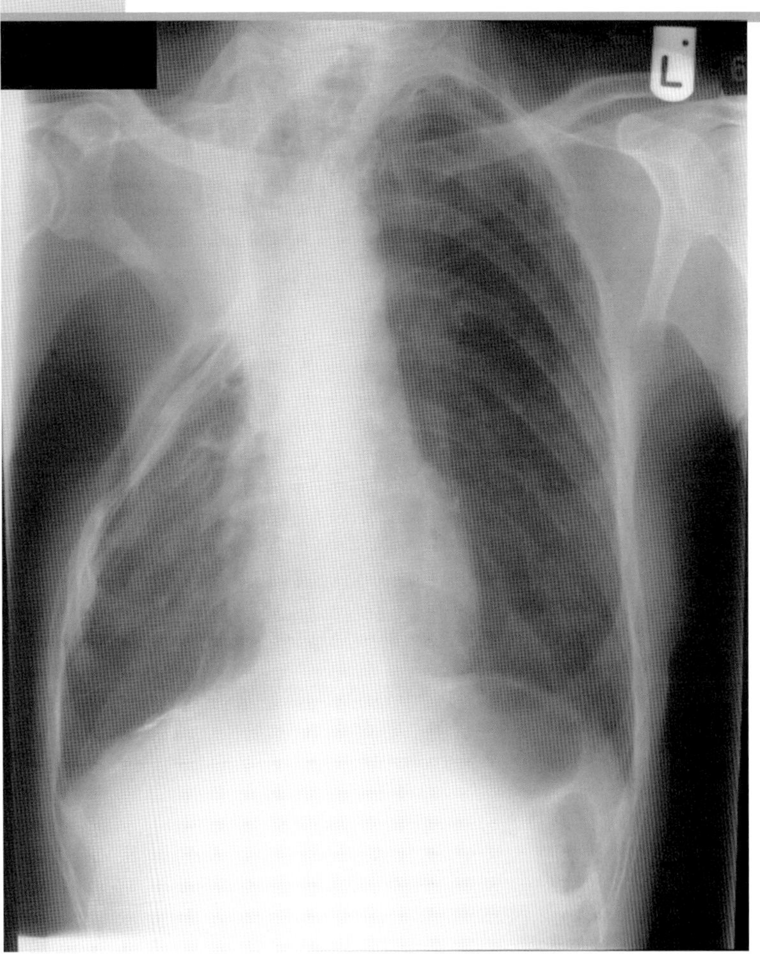

Initial impression

Abnormal chest wall.

Interpretation

This film is obviously abnormal. The right side of the chest looks as if it has been crushed. You cannot see any lung in the upper zone of the right side and the chest wall looks as if it has been pushed against the mediastinum. This appearance is caused by an operation known as thoracoplasty, which used to be a treatment for tuberculosis. It is an appearance you may still come across in elderly patients. A similar film appearance may be seen following trauma.

Notice also the right diaphragm. There is an area of calcification along the diaphragm that may be related to the original tuberculosis.

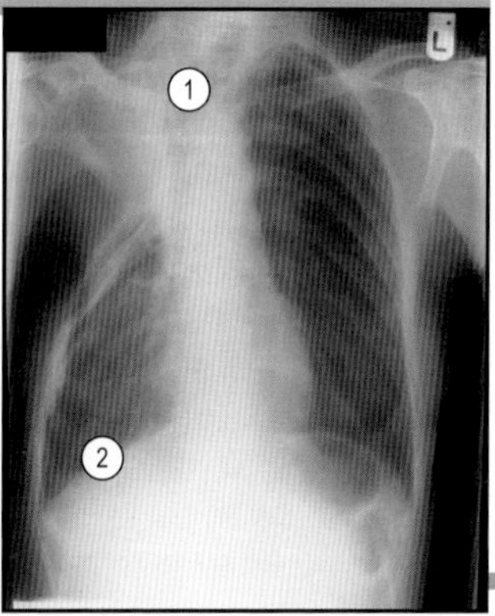

Above: 1. Deviated trachea. 2. Calcification on diaphragm.

SUMMARY

This woman has previously had a right thoracoplasty.

CXR 70

This 80-year-old ex-smoker presented to the emergency department with haemoptysis. What is the most likely diagnosis?

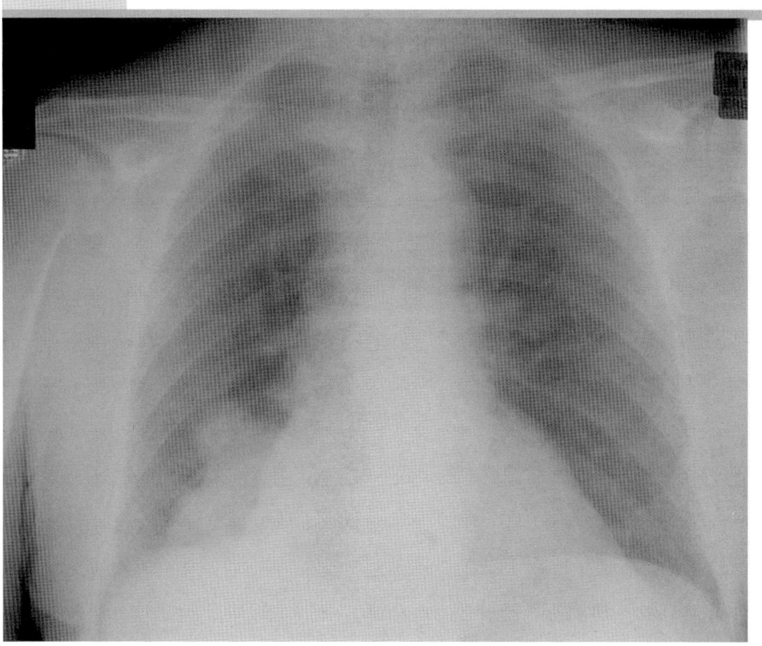

Initial impression

Large white shadow in the right lower zone.

Interpretation

There is a large lobulated mass lesion in the right lower zone. The right heart border is still visible so the mass lesion is not in the middle lobe. The mass can be seen separate from the heart, indicating a posterior location. The right hilum is not bulky and no further lung lesions are seen. The appearances are of a bronchial carcinoma.

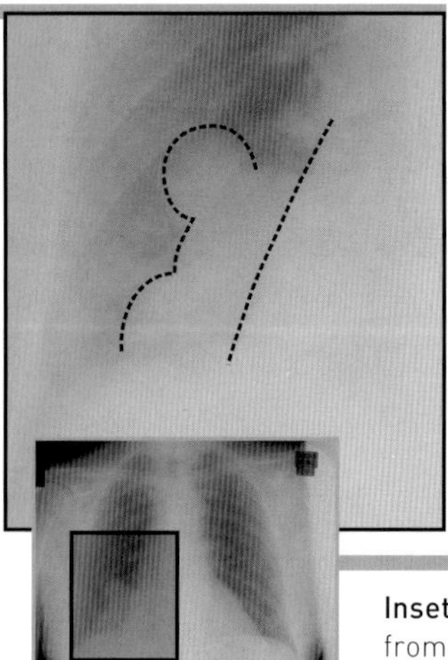

Inset: Lobulated tumour mass is seen separate from the right heart border.

SUMMARY

Large lobulated right lower lobe tumour.

CXR 71

This is the film of a 59-year-old man with a 6-month history of increased shortness of breath. What disease process is suggested by the film appearance?

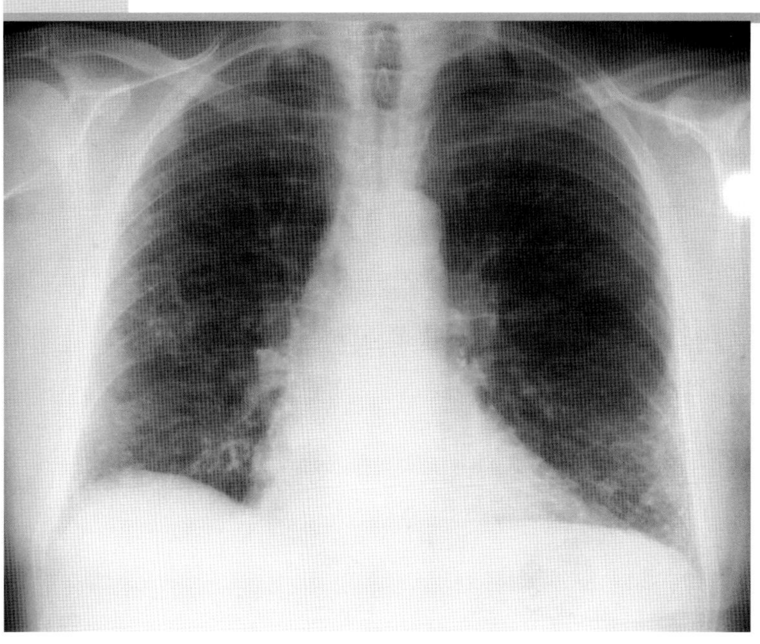

Initial impression

Bilateral white lungs.

Interpretation

The lower zones of both lungs appear whiter than they should. Look at the nature of this whiteness. It is not homogeneous so is unlikely to be either pleural fluid or lung collapse. Instead the whiteness has a mesh-like appearance. This is reticular (net-like) shadowing typical of pulmonary fibrosis.

Look at the distribution of the shadowing. It is most pronounced at the bases and extends into the axillary aspect of each lung. This distribution is commonly seen in cryptogenic fibrosing alveolitis.

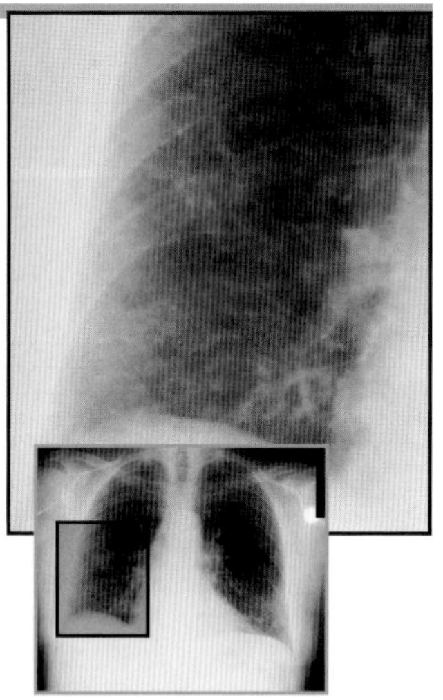

SUMMARY

Cryptogenic fibrosing alveolitis.

CXR 72

This 55-year-old man was recently treated by his GP for pneumonia but failed to respond to antibiotics. He has now completed two courses of antibiotics but continues to have a fever, right-sided chest pains and feels generally unwell. What investigation would you perform next?

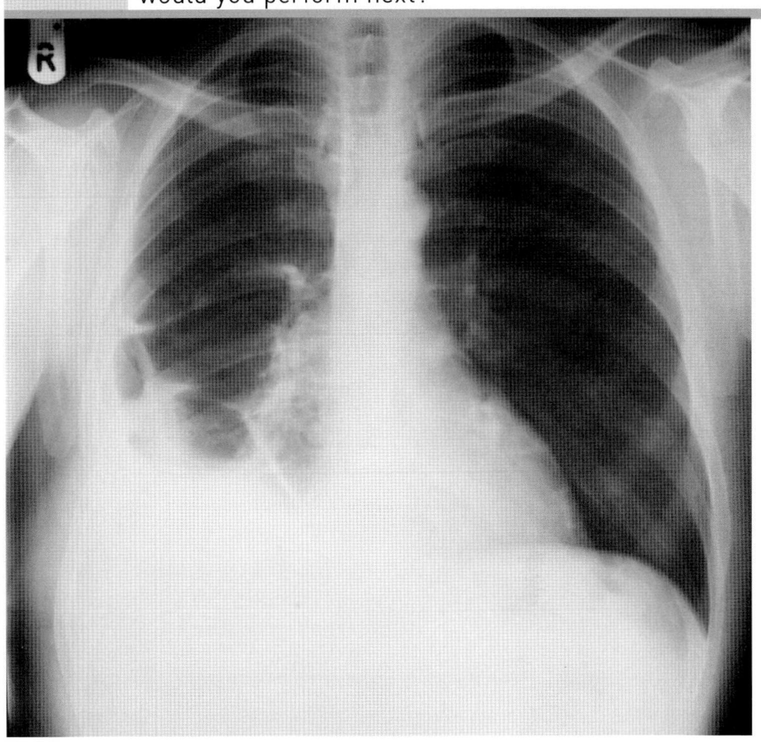

Initial impression

White lung.

Interpretation

Initial survey shows that the abnormality is at the right base. There is a white shadowing that is homogeneous in nature and which obscures the diaphragm and costophrenic angle. There is a meniscus visible laterally. This shadow is due to fluid and in the context of the clinical history is likely to be an empyema.

There are some other white shadows on this film. There is a linear band extending diagonally upwards and outwards from the angle of the heart to the right diaphragm. This is unlikely to be fluid because it does not follow any natural tracts (i.e. any of the fissures). It is linear atelectasis perhaps resulting from the pneumonia. In contrast, the whiteness peripherally on the right (arrow) is fluid tracking up laterally around the fissures. Within this there is an area of increased blackness, indicating gas in the pleural space. This gas may be due to an anaerobic organism, a bronchopleural fistula, or introduced by the medical staff during an aspiration of the empyema.

A diagnostic pleural aspiration (if not already performed!) would be the next investigation in this man.

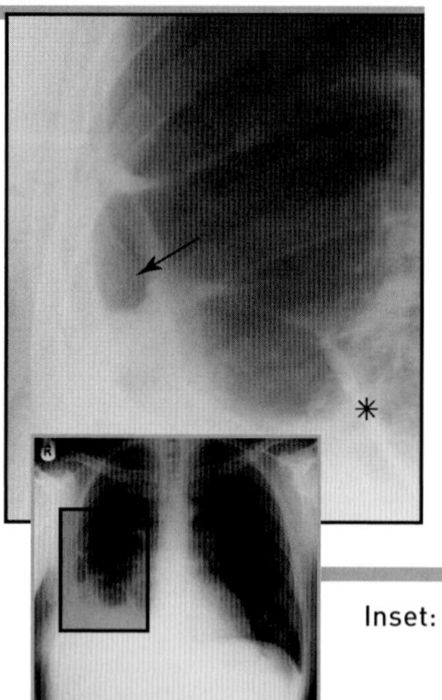

Inset: *Area of atelectasis.

SUMMARY

Pleural fluid with small pockets of gas and linear atelectasis. Probable empyema.

CXR 73

This 60-year-old retired naval officer with a history of asbestos exposure presents with left-sided chest pain. How would you report the film?

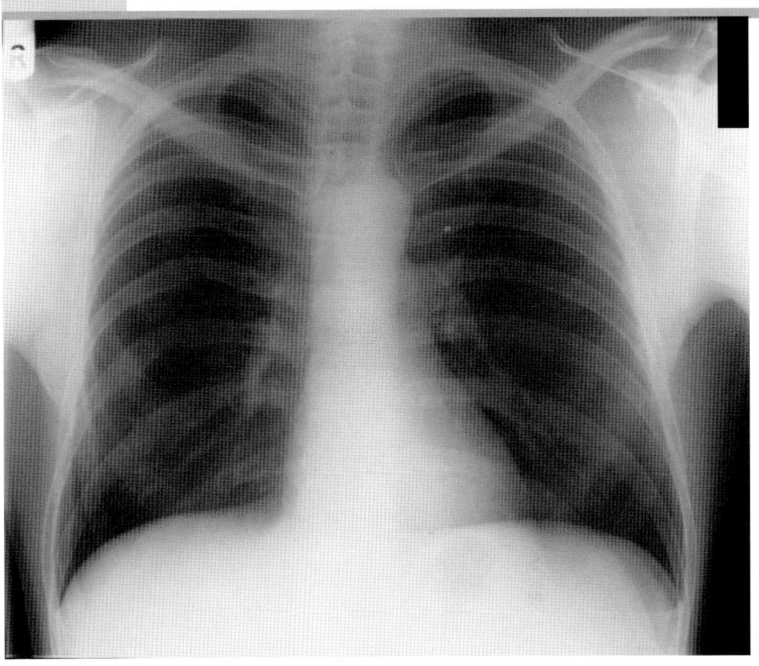

Initial impression

Right-sided rib abnormalities.

Interpretation

Although the film was performed to look for signs of asbestos-related disease there is no evidence of pleural plaques or pleural thickening. The lung fields look normal.

On the right side you can see three rib fractures. You can tell that these are old, healed fractures as the fracture lines are not visible and there is surrounding callus formation. These are in a vertical line involving the posterior right 7th, 8th and 9th ribs. They are therefore most likely to have occurred at the same traumatic incident. This is in contrast to multiple fractures which are found scattered randomly around the chest and that are likely to have occurred from multiple falls, for example in an alcoholic or secondary to bone metastases.

Notice also the metal density overlying the left 6th rib posteriorly. This cannot be localized further on a PA film and is probably an artefact.

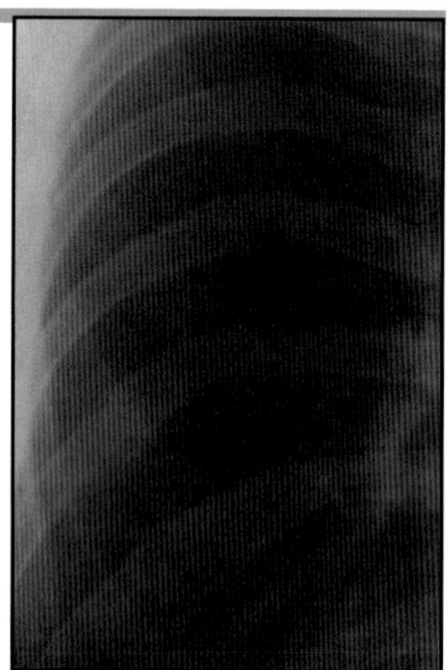

SUMMARY

Three old right rib fractures. Metal artefact over left chest.

CXR 74

This is the film of a 45-year-old woman with a known history of breast cancer, which was treated with mastectomy and chemotherapy. She presented to her GP with a persistent dry cough. What does the film show?

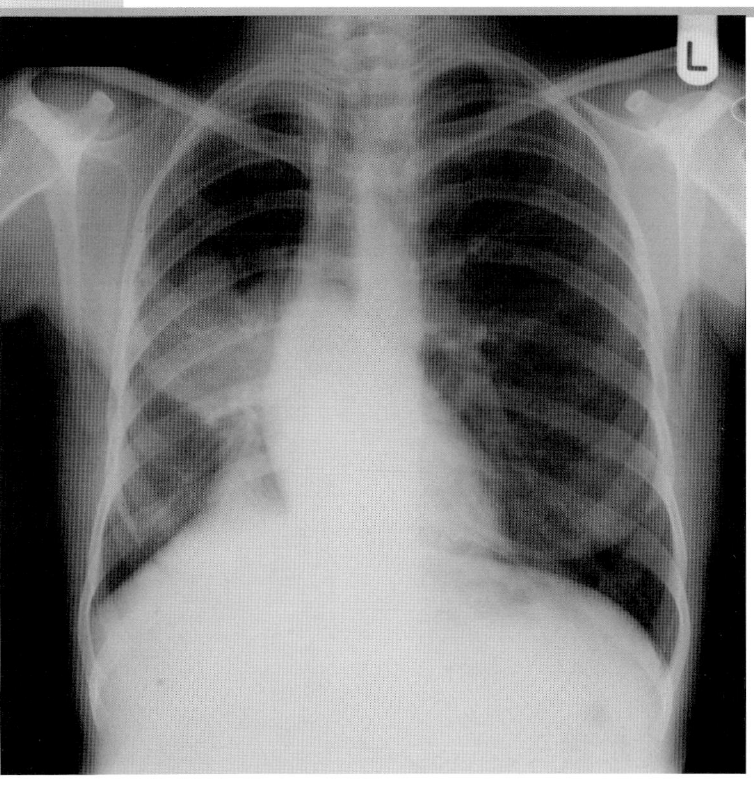

Initial impression

Abnormal white lung in the right mid zone.

Interpretation

There is an abnormal area of white lung in the right mid zone. Look carefully at the right lung and you will see a number of clues suggesting that this is due to an area of lung collapse. Look at the position of the trachea and note how it has been pulled to the right. This suggests loss of volume on the right side. Look carefully at the right hemidiaphragm. There has been distortion of the right hemidiaphragm and loss of clarity at its most medial end. In contrast, the right heart border is clearly seen. This is important in differentiating right lower lobe and right middle lobe collapse – the right lower lobe will collapse against the diaphragm, giving it an indistinct appearance on film, whereas the right middle lobe will collapse against the heart, giving an indistinct right heart border. This film shows right lower lobe collapse due, in this case, to a right mid zone lung mass, which is invading the right main bronchus and causing the lower lobe collapse.

Always remember to complete your survey of the film by examining the soft tissues, which in this case gives you important information. You will notice asymmetry of the breast shadows, and the curvilinear lower border is lost on the right. The left axilla has normal margins, but they are distorted on the right. Both these changes reflect the mastectomy.

SUMMARY

Right mastectomy. Intrapulmonary mass at the right hilum likely to be metastasis from previous breast cancer, causing right lower lobe collapse.

CXR 75

This is a lateral film from an earlier study, showing a left-sided abnormality. Can you identify what the abnormality is from the film?

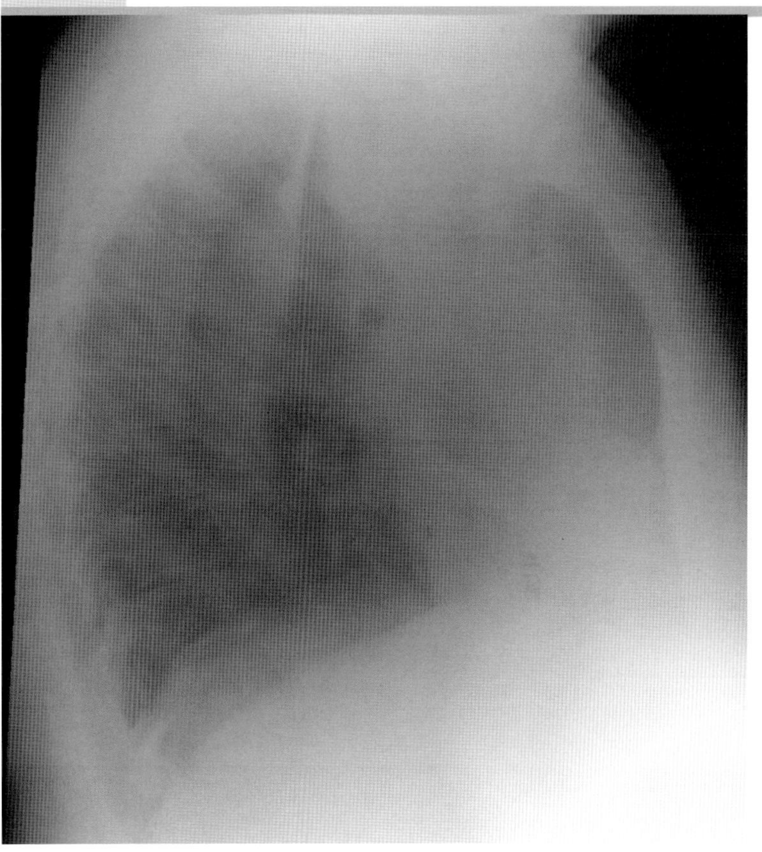

Initial impression

Increased white density at the front of the chest.

Interpretation

Remember the guide to interpreting the lateral film.

In this study, neither diaphragm is elevated. There are, however, two important abnormalities. The first is the increased density seen behind the sternum – there is in-filling of the retro-sternal window, which should normally be the darkest part of the film. This implies that there is an abnormality lying anteriorly, increasing the density here. The second abnormality is the oblique density running from the top of the chest from around the second thoracic vertebra, to near the anterior chest wall. The density is lost over the mid cardiac region. The oblique fissure is often visible on a lateral film, and this would run from the level of T4/5 posteriorly to the proximal third of the diaphragm anteriorly. The density we are seeing represents a displaced oblique fissure, which has moved forwards as the lung collapses, and the increased density within the collapsed-down lung has caused the whiteness in the retro-sternal window.

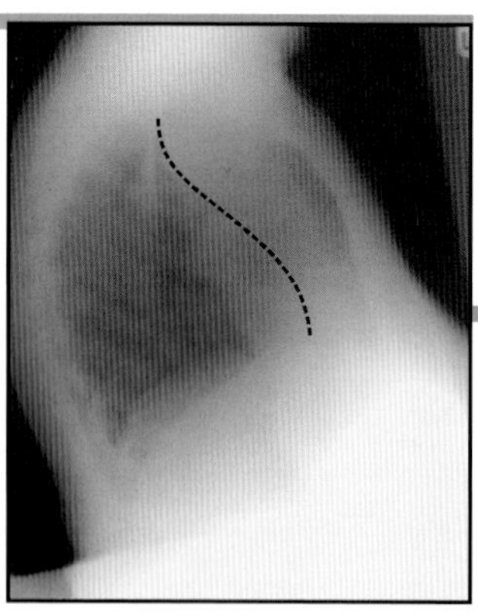

An endoluminal tumour of a proximal upper lobe bronchus should be investigated for.

Left: Oblique fissure pulled forwards as a result of the upper lobe collapse.

SUMMARY

Upper lobe collapse.

CXR 76

This is the film of an 82-year-old woman with weight loss and a long history of a productive cough. What does the film show?

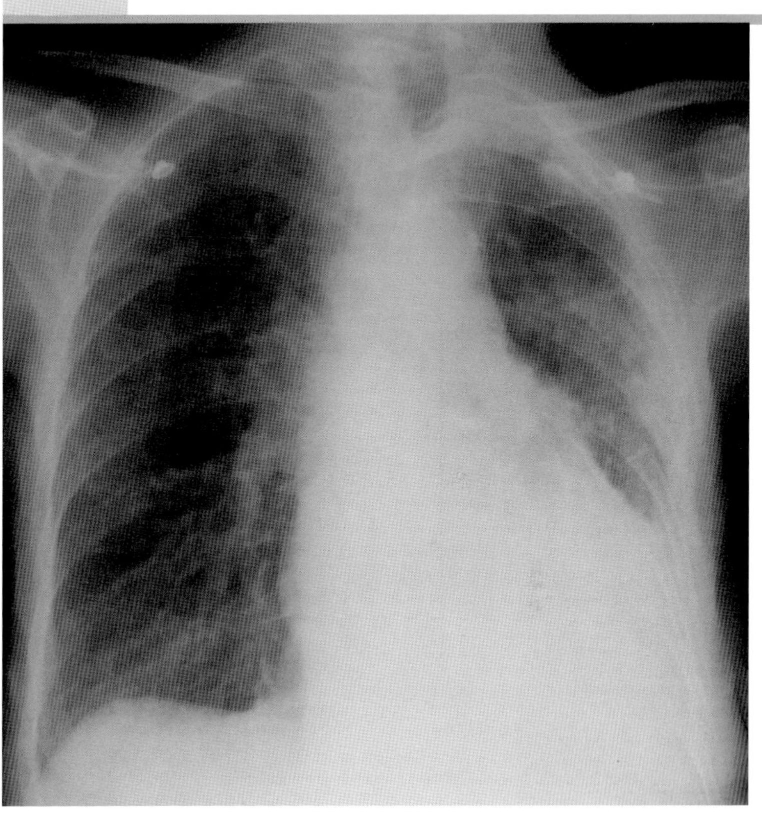

Initial impression

Thin woman with white lungs.

Interpretation

There is a paucity of soft tissue shadows around the chest and shoulder girdle indicating a thin, wasted patient. The lung fields are white. The cause for this whiteness can be most clearly seen at the right lower zone. Here you can see parallel thickened white lines and occasional round shadows, which are the tramlines and ring shadows of bronchiectasis. Chronic bronchiectasis would be the cause of this person's wasted appearance.

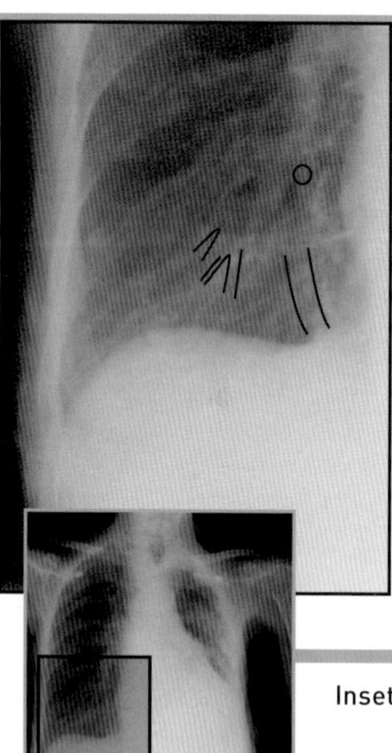

Inset: Ring shadows and tram lines (see CXR 43).

SUMMARY

Bronchiectasis.

CXR 77

This is the film of a 51-year-old man. His GP ordered it after the patient complained of a persistent cough. What is the subtle (incidental) finding?

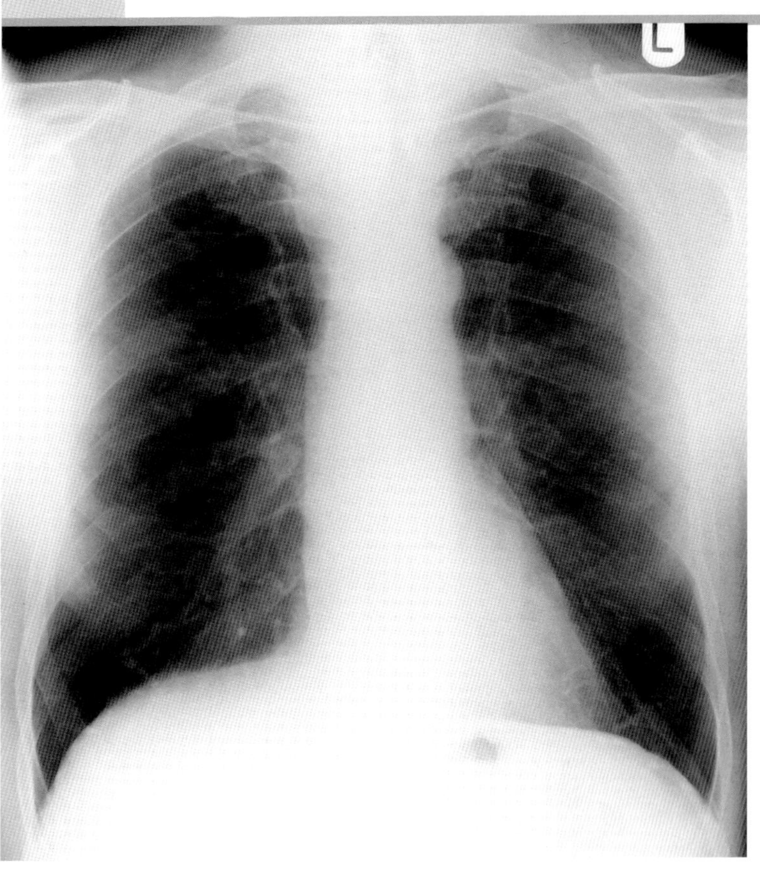

Initial impression

Abnormal mediastinum.

Interpretation

The abnormality on this film is subtle. However, if you look carefully at the mediastinum you will notice increased density and some widening of the upper part. There are no defined limits to the width of the mediastinum so deciding whether it is widened or not is a matter of experience.

If you suspect a widening of the mediastinum then you need to think about its possible cause. First decide which part is widened. A widening of the upper part could be due to abnormalities of the thyroid, thymus or innominate artery. Abnormalities in the middle or lower part of the mediastinum could be due to a widened aorta, lymphadenopathy, dilatation of the oesophagus or hiatus hernia.

In this film it is the top of the mediastinum that is widened. This narrows the pathology down to the thyroid, thymus or innominate artery. Look at the area at the top of the mediastinum where the thyroid normally sits. Look also at the effect on other mediastinal structures. The thyroid is in the same compartment as the trachea. Therefore, if you suspect thyroid enlargement, look carefully at the trachea since this may either be displaced or (less commonly) narrowed by thyroid enlargement. In this film the trachea has been pushed to the left, making thyroid enlargement the most likely diagnosis.

SUMMARY

Thyroid enlargement, likely to be benign.

CXR 78

This is the film of a 52-year-old woman who was admitted through the emergency department with a 1-day history of profound shortness of breath. She smoked 10 cigarettes per day but had previously been fit and well. What is the most likely diagnosis? Is a follow-up film necessary?

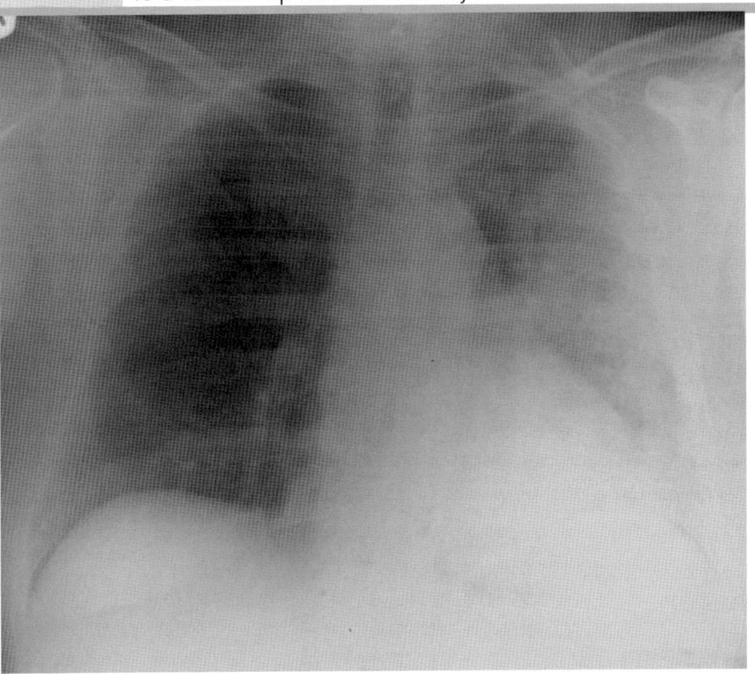

Initial impression

Abnormal white shadow in the left lung.

Interpretation

There is an area of whiteness in the left lung field. The shadowing is not homogeneous in nature. Look closely at the shadowing and you will see an air bronchogram, i.e. the bronchi appear as black thick lines within the white shadow. The carina remains central, and the volume of the underlying lung looks well preserved, so there is unlikely to be any associated collapse. An air bronchogram suggests the presence of consolidation and this is most likely to indicate left lower lobe pneumonia.

The changes of pneumonia often take 6 weeks to resolve and persistent change can indicate the presence of an obstructing neoplasm. This woman is at risk of a bronchial carcinoma since she is over 40 and a smoker. The film should therefore be repeated in 6 weeks to ensure the area of infection is resolving. If there were no significant improvement the patient should undergo further investigation, by bronchoscopy or CT scan to identify or exclude any underlying neoplasm. In this case, the follow-up film at 6 weeks did show total clearing of the consolidation.

SUMMARY

Area of consolidation due to pneumonia. Follow-up film needed at 6 weeks.

CXR 79

This is the film of a 77-year-old woman who presented following two episodes of haemoptysis. What is the abnormality and how would you investigate further?

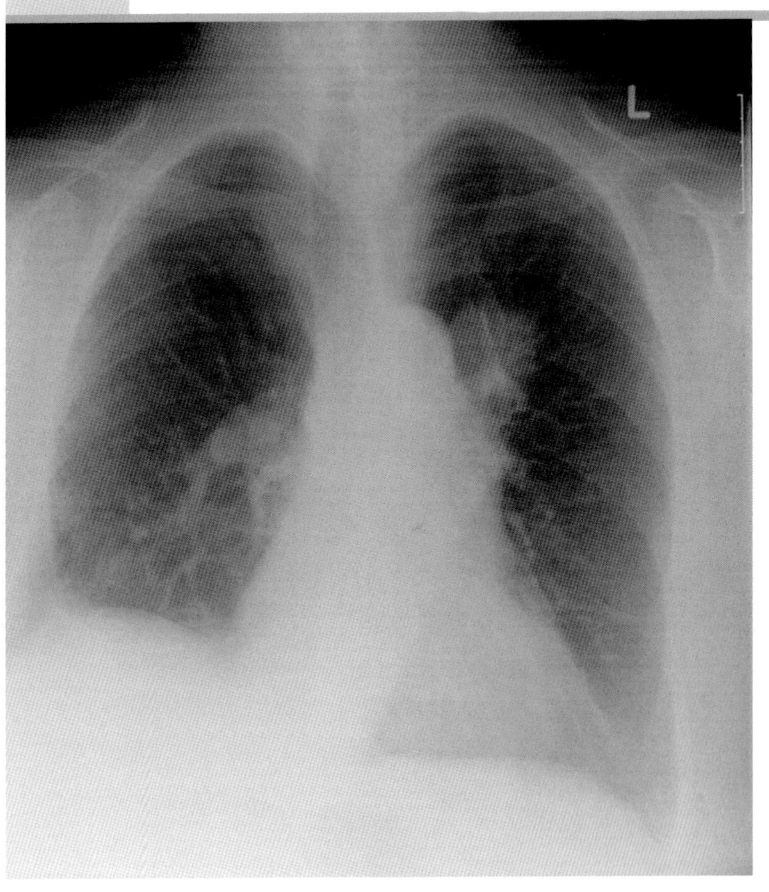

Initial impression

Abnormally shaped left hilum.

Interpretation

There is a rounded white lesion above the left hilum and the pulmonary artery can be seen separately from this. The upper outer margin of the lesion is irregular. There is a thoracic scoliosis concave to the right. This is a common feature on chest films in the elderly, and rib crowding, mediastinal distortion and lung volume changes can be seen as a result. No other lesions or areas of bone destruction are seen. The irregular appearance of this lesion is suggestive of malignancy. A bronchoscopy and staging CT scan would be the most appropriate next investigation.

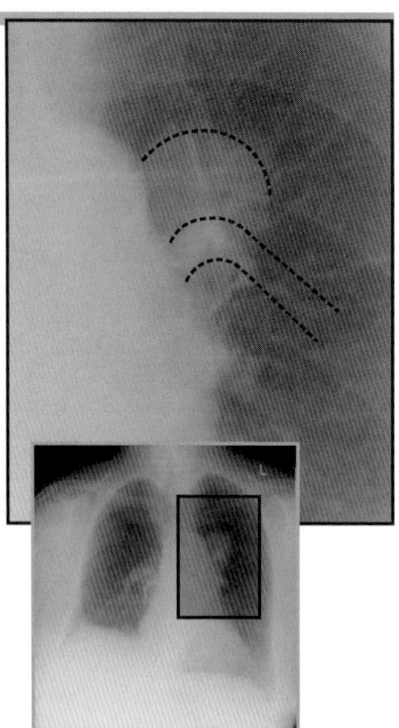

SUMMARY

Probable lung malignancy.

CXR 80

This is the film of a 48-year-old Algerian taken when he applied for immigration to the UK. What does it show?

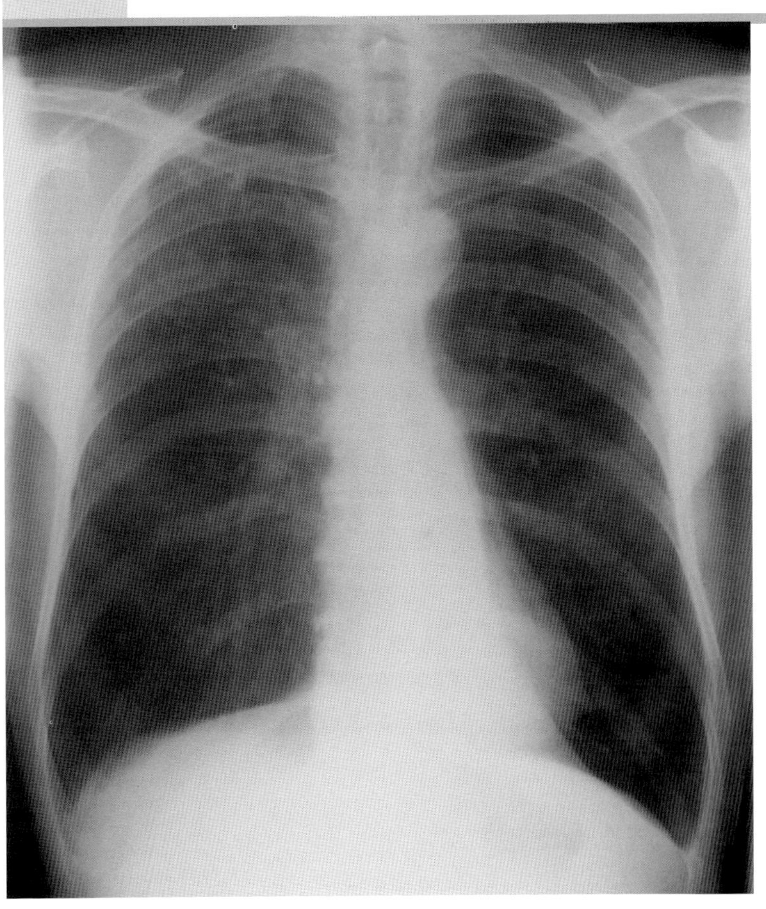

Initial impression

Area of whiteness in the right upper zone.

Interpretation

There is an area of whiteness in the right upper zone. On looking closely you can see that this is made up of lots of small nodules. The nature and the upper zone distribution would suggest tuberculosis. This may be scarring from previous disease as some areas are very dense, suggesting calcification, but an active form should also be considered.

Always remember to view the whole of the film and not to stop the search after identifying the first abnormality. Study of this film shows a triangular area of dense whiteness behind the heart shadow. The margin of the left hemidiaphragm is obscured medially, and there is some shift of the heart border, as the right side of the vertebral bodies can be seen more clearly than usual. This is the typical appearance of left lower lobe collapse. The lower lobe may be collapsed by an endoluminal blockage, or by damage to the wall of the lower lobe bronchus by tuberculosis.

It can be difficult to distinguish current from old tuberculosis. The presence of lung or pleural calcification can suggest old disease, and it is also helpful to compare with previous films, or perform follow-up films to look for disease progression. Obviously the clinical context is extremely important.

SUMMARY

Old tuberculosis and left lower lobe collapse.

CXR 81

A 74-year-old man presented to his GP with a 2-month history of weight loss and fatigue. He also complained of pain in his right shoulder and down the inner surface of his arm. On examination the GP noticed that his right pupil was abnormally constricted. What does this film demonstrate?

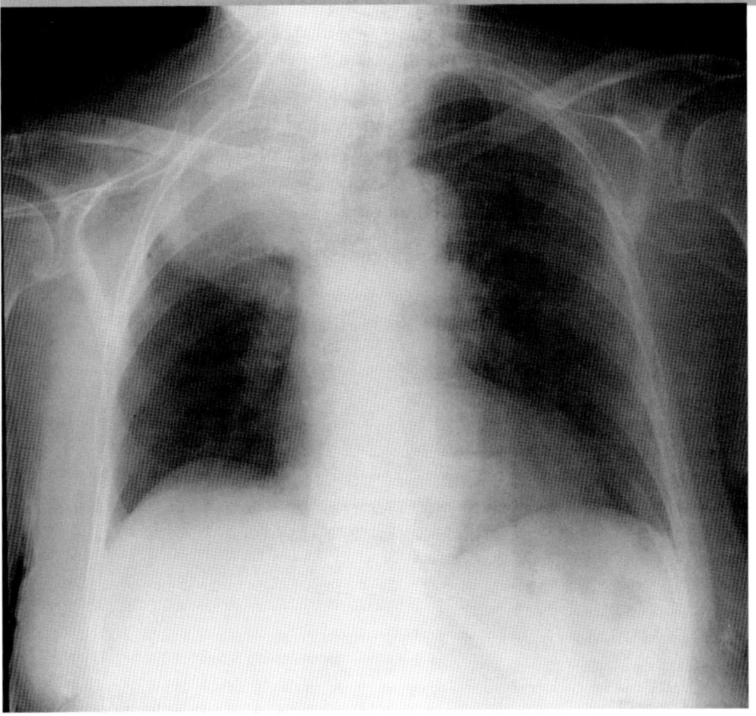

Initial impression

Abnormal whiteness of the right upper zone.

Interpretation

The increased whiteness in the right upper zone does not appear to contain any bronchograms. The lower border is curved. Look carefully at the margin of the first rib and you can see that the posterior portion of the rib has been destroyed. The history and these features suggest a malignant process. The abnormal neurological findings are those of involvement of the brachial plexus, and the outflow of the cervical sympathetic nerves.

This is a Pancoast tumour.

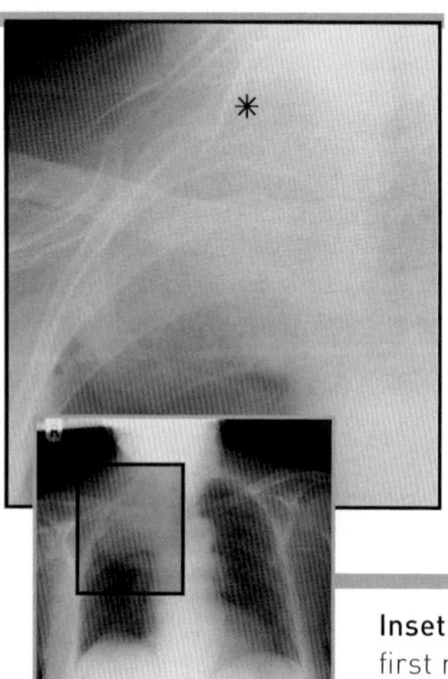

Inset: Asterisk shows position of destroyed first rib.

SUMMARY

Right apical mass with bone destruction. Pancoast tumour.

CXR 82

Why is this 58-year-old woman short of breath?

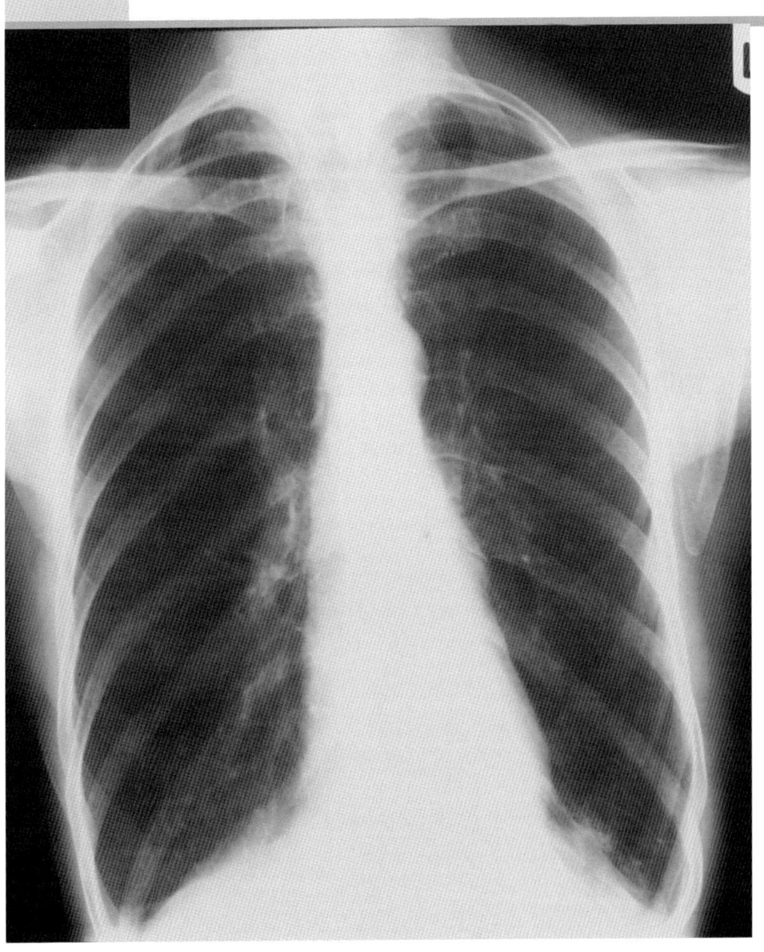

Initial impression

Large black lungs.

Interpretation

The most obvious abnormality is the black lung fields. Black lung can be caused by over-penetration, emphysema, pneumothorax or, rarely, massive pulmonary embolus. This film is not over-penetrated. The fact that both lungs are black means that this patient is likely to have emphysema.

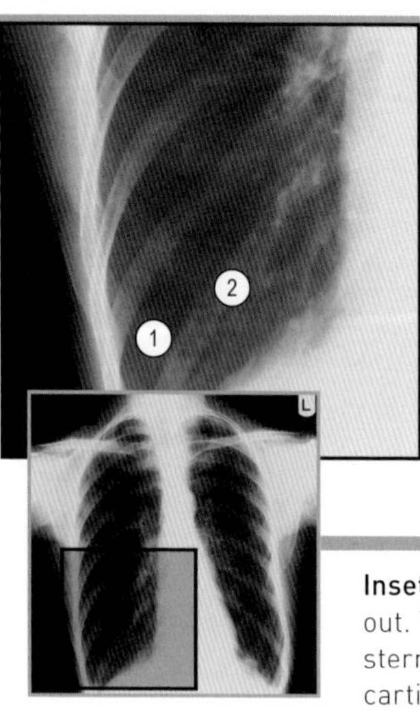

This film demonstrates a number of features consistent with emphysema. You can count more than seven ribs anteriorly, which indicates that the lung fields are large. The heart and mediastinum are long and thin and the diaphragms appear flattened. These are also signs of a hyperexpanded thorax. As is often the case in severe emphysema there is such widespread emphysematous changes that you cannot identify individual bullae.

Inset: 1. Anterior ribs often appear to end by fading out. They connect via costal cartilage to the sternum. The degree of calcification in the cartilage varies between individuals and increases with age. 2. Posterior ribs extend medially to the vertebral columns.

SUMMARY

Chronic obstructive pulmonary disease.

CXR 83

This is the film of a 52-year-old woman with chronic shortness of breath. She has never smoked. Are there any clues from the film as to the cause of her breathlessness?

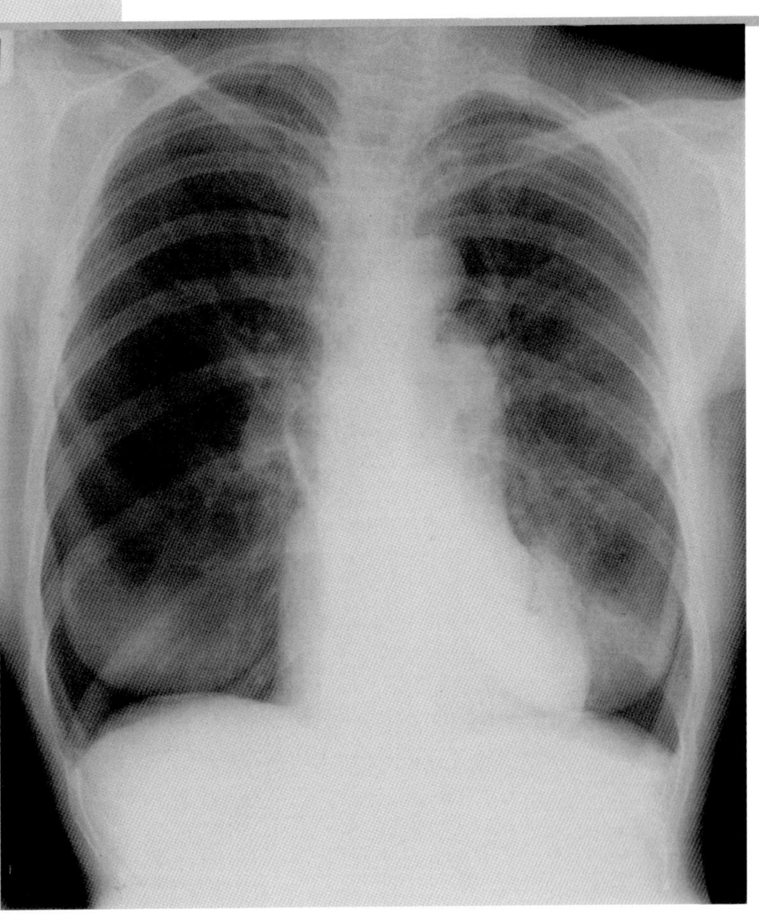

Initial impression

Normal film.

Interpretation

There is nothing obvious on the film. Therefore you need to look carefully at the areas where abnormalities can easily be missed – the apices, behind the heart and under the diaphragm. If these areas are normal then look for signs of a small pneumothorax. In this film, these areas look normal and there is no evidence of a small pneumothorax.

Another area where subtle differences in lung density can be missed is the lower zone, where the lungs are partially obscured by the breast shadows. In this film these areas look abnormally black. This is due to an absence of vascular markings within the lungs. Confirm this by looking at the right hilum and try to identify the lower lobe pulmonary artery. It is difficult to see and the right hilum appears truncated at the lower part. The left hilum may well be similar, but is obscured by the heart shadow.

These features suggest lower zone emphysema. If you detect lower zone, as opposed to upper zone, emphysema then you must think of alpha-1 antitrypsin deficiency and, in this case, this would fit with the clinical history of emphysema in a 52-year-old who has never smoked. A CT scan confirmed the presence of bilateral mid to lower zone emphysema. This is the reverse pattern to smoking-related emphysema, which predominantly affects the upper zones.

SUMMARY

Lower zone emphysema, secondary to alpha-1 antitrypsin deficiency.

CXR 84

This 68-year-old woman presented with a history of increasing breathlessness on exertion and orthopnoea. What is the likely cause of her symptoms?

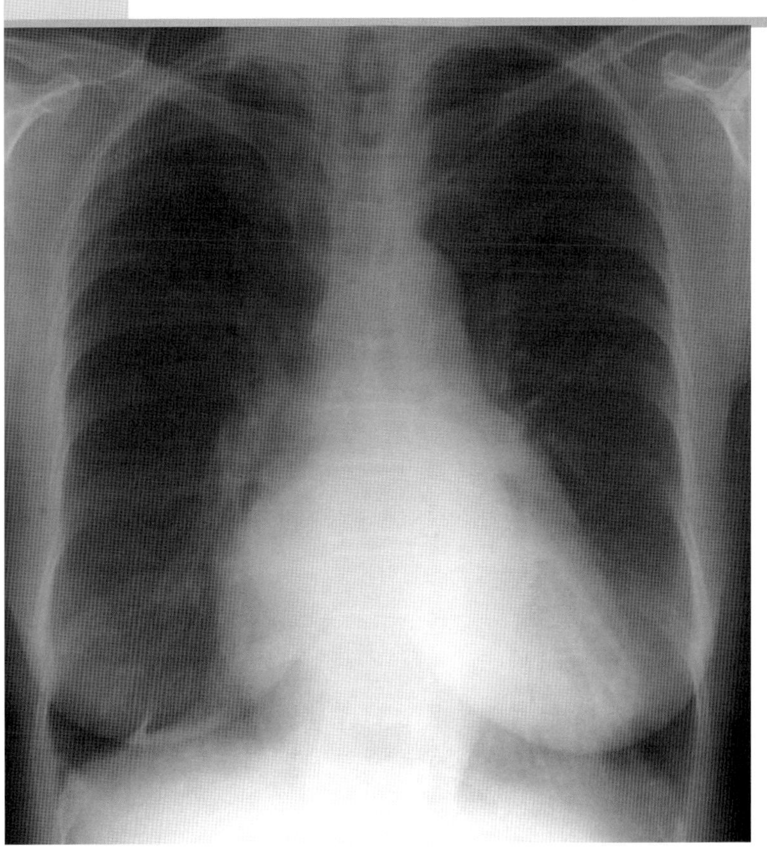

Initial impression

Abnormal heart shadow.

Interpretation

The heart is enlarged as it is more than half the diameter of the chest. Look carefully at the shape of the heart. The enlarged area is mainly to the right of the midline rather than to the left. This part of the heart is made up of the left and right atrium so one of these structures must be enlarged. There is an increased rounded density centred on the midline, and the proximal left and right main bronchi are pushed apart. You can tell this because the angle between the left and right main bronchus is more than 90°. The area of the heart between the left and right main bronchus is the left atrium. This woman has left atrial enlargement.

Left atrial enlargement is seen in mitral valve disease. A regurgitant mitral valve would put a volume load on the left ventricle, which may result in enlargement of the ventricle to the left of the midline. A stenotic valve does not volume load the left ventricle. There is no evidence of left ventricular enlargement on this film and this woman is therefore more likely to have mitral stenosis.

There is some linear scarring at the right lung base. This is due to atelectasis of the lung.

SUMMARY

This woman's symptoms are due to mitral stenosis.

CXR 85

This 55-year-old woman presented to the acute medical admissions unit with a 3-week history of haemoptysis. What does her film show?

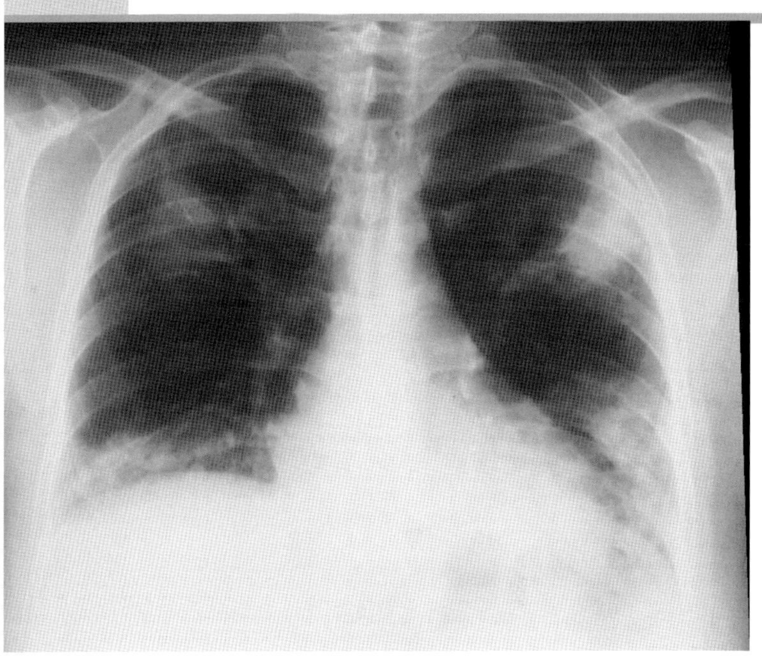

Initial impression

Multiple peripheral white shadows.

Interpretation

There are only 5 anterior ribs visible on the chest film, indicating poor inspiration. This sometimes indicates that the patient is too breathless to take an adequate breath in.

There are bilateral peripheral white shadows with poorly defined margins. They are all of different sizes.

The film shows multiple ill-defined lesions. The differential diagnosis is quite broad and would include multiple metastases, blood-borne infections, pulmonary infarcts, vasculitic lesions and cryptogenic causes. A number of idiopathic conditions, such as eosinophilic pneumonia, or cryptogenic organizing pneumonia, are characterized by multiple lung shadows but cavitation is not a feature. Pulmonary metastases often have well-defined margins, which is not the case in this film. The lesions are quite large for a multifocal infection and the clinical history is not typical for acute infection. Pulmonary infarcts of this size would be unusual.

The diagnosis here was a vasculitis – Wegener's granulomatosis. There was accompanying renal involvement, and diagnosis was confirmed on renal biopsy.

SUMMARY

Bilateral multifocal areas of consolidation, at biopsy proven to be secondary to Wegener's granulomatosis.

CXR 86

This 77-year-old woman presented to the emergency department of her local hospital with a 3-month history of retrosternal chest pain radiating through to her back. She presented when the pain suddenly got worse. How would you interpret the film?

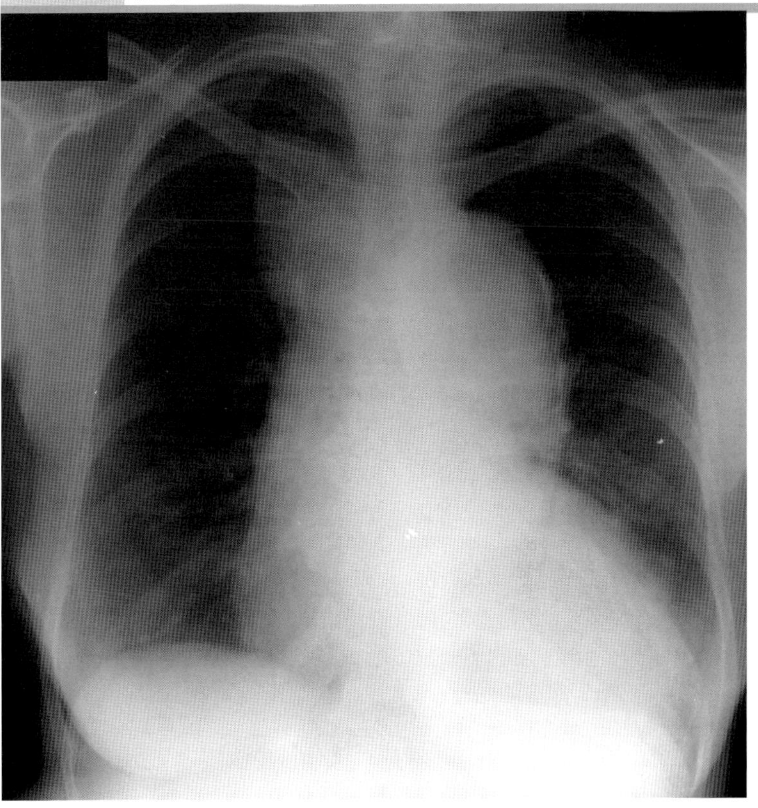

Initial impression

Abnormal white mediastinum and large heart.

Interpretation

The heart is enlarged as it takes up more than half the cardiothoracic diameter. The mediastinum is also widened. You now need to decide which part of the mediastinum is widened. The area above the clavicles either side of the trachea is normal, so the upper part of the mediastinum, which contains the thyroid, is normal. The middle part of the mediastinum, just under the clavicles, contains the aorta, pulmonary artery and mediastinal lymph nodes. This is the part that is widened on this film.

You need to decide which structure has caused the widened appearance. It is difficult to determine this by the shape of the mediastinum. Look for the aortic shadow. If the aorta was the cause of the enlargement you would not expect to see a separate aortic shadow. This is the case in this film, where a separate aortic shadow is not visible. Another clue is the presence of a line of calcium curved around the left margin of the enlarged area. This is calcification of the vessel wall. This appears different from lymph node calcification where the line of calcium is generally smaller and more circular. This patient had a fusiform aneurysm of the ascending aorta, which was the cause of her chest and back pain.

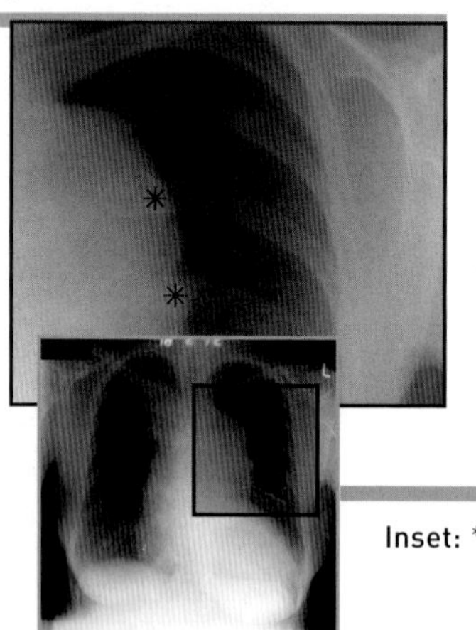

Inset: *Small areas of aortic wall calcification.

SUMMARY

Fusiform aortic aneurysm.

CXR 87

This 63-year-old clerical officer gave a long history of cough and shortness of breath. What does the film show?

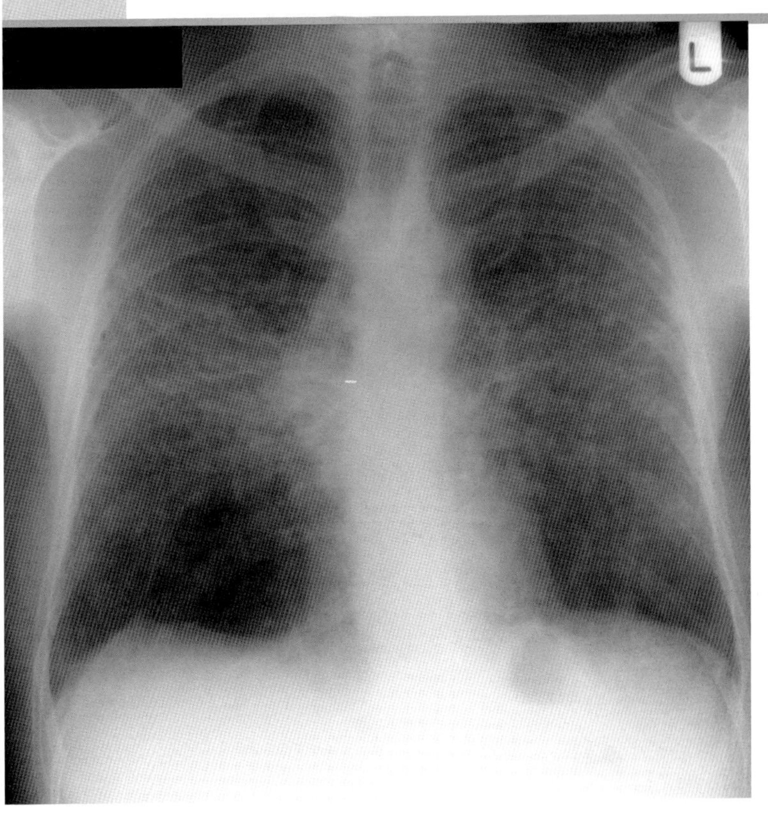

Initial impression

Bilateral white lungs.

Interpretation

Both lungs are whiter than they should be. Look at the distribution and nature of the whiteness. The whiteness is most marked in the mid zones of both lungs. The whiteness is streaky in nature. The hilar are distorted and appear to have been pulled out by the shadowing. The distribution of the shadowing suggests sarcoidosis and the distortion of the hilar indicate a fibrotic process – the fibrous tissue contracting the lung and pulling on the hila.

Do not be put off by the absence of a honeycombing pattern. Although honeycombing often occurs with fibrosis this is not always the case. In this film it is the streaky nature of the shadowing and lung distortion that suggest pulmonary fibrosis.

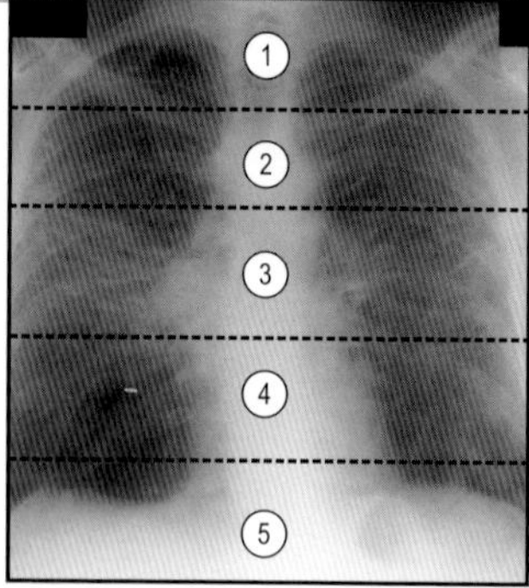

Above: 1. Apices. 2. Upper zones. 3. Mid zones. 4. Lower zones. 5. Bases.

SUMMARY

Upper and mid zone fibrosis secondary to sarcoidosis.

CXR 88

This 75-year-old man developed severe constant pain on the left side of his chest that initially responded well to non-steroidal anti-inflammatory medication. He was persuaded to see his GP by his neighbour who was worried because he had had the pain for over 2 months. The GP organized a film and referred him immediately to the local chest clinic. What does this film show?

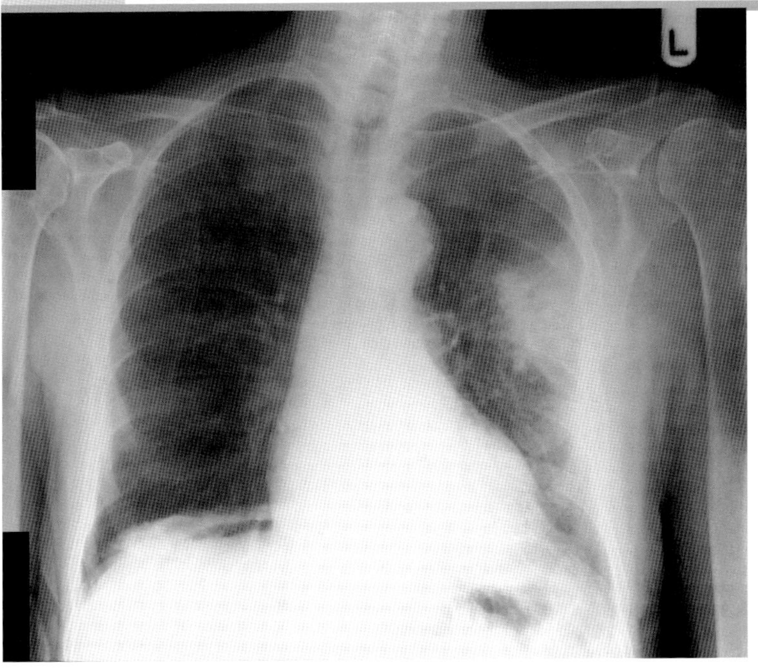

Initial impression

Whiteness of the left lung.

Interpretation

There is a white shadow located in the peripheral part of the left mid zone. The shadowing is homogeneous in nature, but has an irregular border. This could be a mass lesion or an area of consolidation. Look for an air bronchogram. There is no air bronchogram present, which goes against consolidation. This is likely to be a mass lesion. Look carefully at the overlying ribs and follow each rib anteriorly from its posterior end. If you do this you will notice that it is not possible to follow the 5th and 6th ribs. This is because they have been destroyed by the aggressive nature of the mass, which is therefore highly likely to be malignant. This man was found to have an adenocarcinoma.

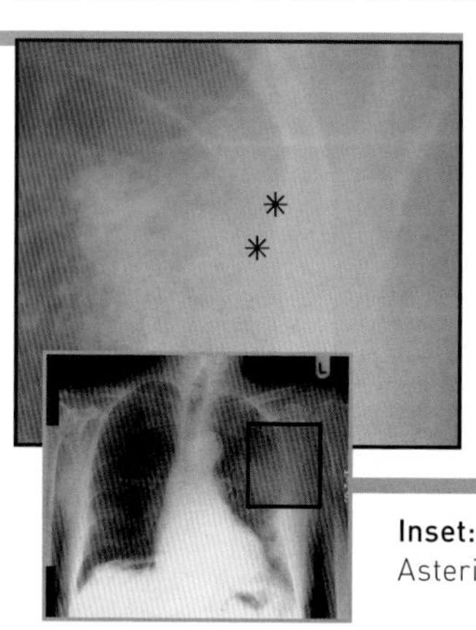

Notice also a rim of blackness underneath the right diaphragm. This is air contained within bowel loops lying in front of and slightly higher than the upper border of the liver.

Inset: The normal rib edge has been destroyed. Asterisks mark position of destroyed rib edge.

SUMMARY

Peripheral malignant lung mass with rib destruction.

CXR 89

This 70-year-old woman gave a 2-month history of small amounts of haemoptysis and a 1-year history of weight loss. She was sent to the chest clinic by her GP for further investigation and this film was taken on her arrival. How would you report the film?

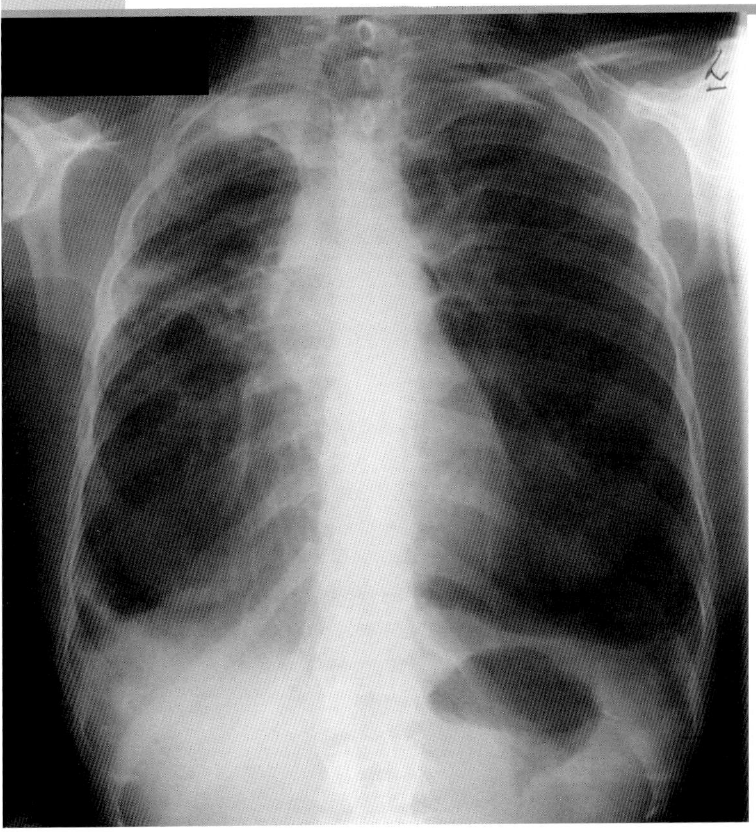

Initial impression

Very thin patient, hila pulled up and apical whiteness.

Interpretation

Although this patient is a woman, the breast shadows are less obvious than usual, which indicates low body weight. This is supported by the absence of subcutaneous fat, which is best appreciated by looking around the lower ribs.

Initial survey of the lung fields shows that both hila have been pulled upwards towards the apex, which is the result of marked volume loss in the upper lobes. Careful examination of the upper zones shows pleural thickening. Tuberculosis is the most common cause of this picture. This woman had *Mycobacterium malmoense*, an atypical mycobacterium, which explains the indolent nature of this disease.

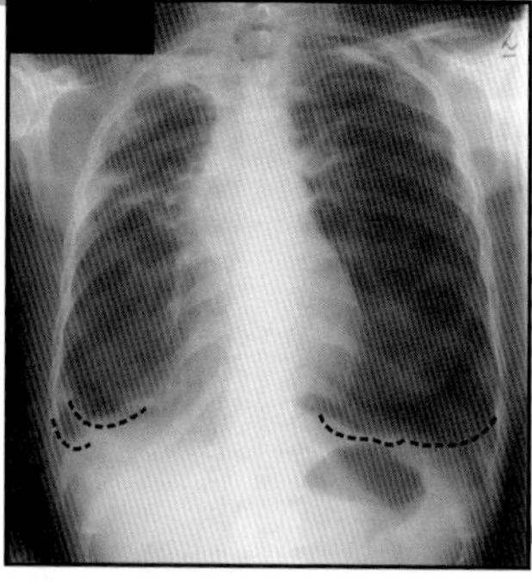

Above: Note scalloping of the diaphragms, a scooped-out appearance seen where the lung is hyperinflated, in this case as compensation for the apical and upper zones' volume loss. This is also seen in emphysema.

SUMMARY

Absence of subcutaneous fat and breast tissue, loss of volume in the upper lobes and apical pleural thickening due to *Mycobacterium malmoense*.

CXR 90

This 76-year-old woman had this film taken because of increasing shortness of breath and a productive cough. What operation has she had in the past and what is the cause of her shortness of breath?

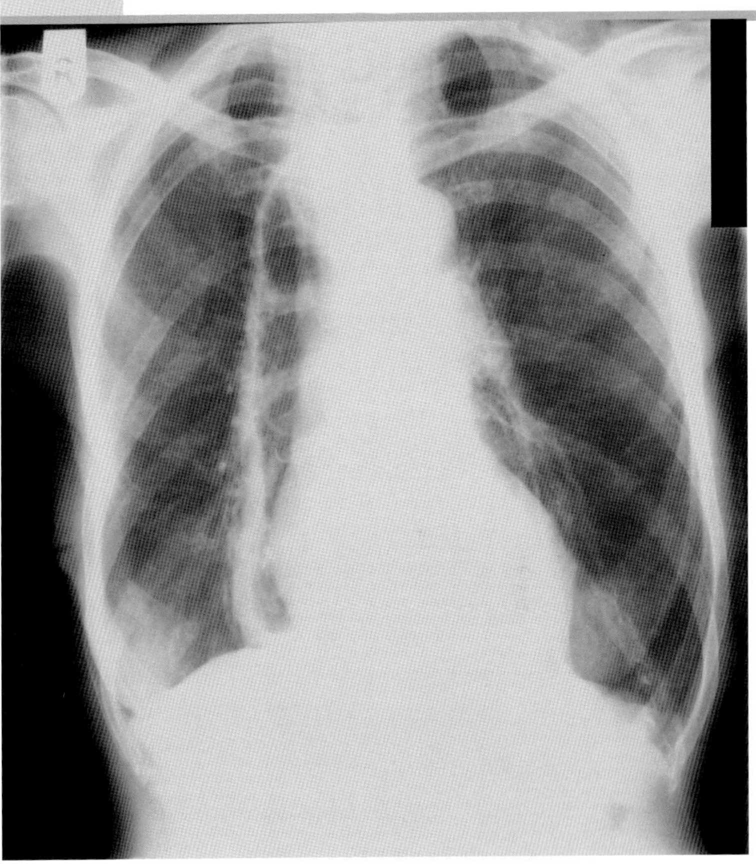

Initial impression

Abnormal white line on the right of the mediastinum.

Interpretation

This is a difficult film, which shows the importance of surveying the whole film to reach a diagnosis.

First look at the abnormal line. It traverses all the lobes of the lung so is unlikely to be a pulmonary or pleural abnormality since it does not follow the pulmonary anatomy. It roughly follows the line of the mediastinum, which makes a mediastinal abnormality more likely. This could be air within the mediastinum, for example a pneumomediastinum or pneumopericardium. Look at the position of the air and the nature of the line. The air goes above the aorta, meaning that this is not a pneumopericardium. The line is very thick, far thicker than the mediastinal pleura, so a simple pneumomediastinum is unlikely. Look at the rest of the film for other clues. When you survey the bones you will see that the right 6th rib is abnormal. As you follow it the contour of the rib disappears. This would suggest that this woman has had a thoracotomy. In fact, this woman had an oesophagectomy 8 years before this film was taken. This involves a gastric pull-up, in which the stomach is pulled up into the chest. The thick white line is the wall of the air-filled stomach outlined by the adjacent lung.

Note also that this woman has large lungs, flat hemidiaphragms and black lungs, especially in the apices. The cause of her breathlessness is chronic obstructive pulmonary disease.

SUMMARY

Previous oesophagectomy and COPD.

CXR 91

This patient has myeloma. What complications can you see on the film?

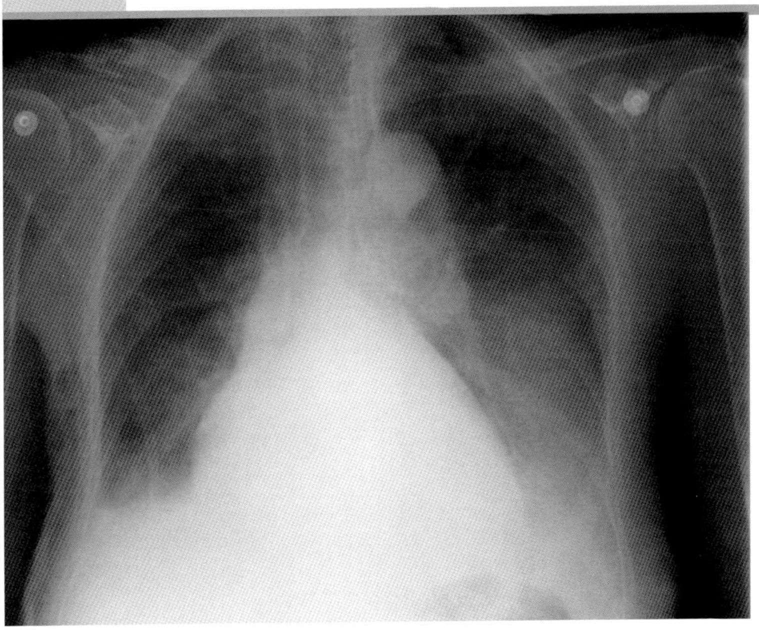

Initial impression

Abnormal white lungs.

Interpretation

Although there is an obvious abnormality in the lungs, this film demonstrates the importance of fully surveying the film.

First note that the film is AP. This suggests that the patient is unwell and also means that limited information can be gained about the heart size. Look at the lung fields. The right diaphragm is completely obscured with loss of the costophrenic angle, which suggests the presence of a pleural effusion. Look at the area of whiteness on the left. This extends from the mid zone down to the base and is hazy in appearance. Look at the diaphragms. The left diaphragm is also obscured by the hazy shadowing on the left lung. The distribution of the left-sided shadowing makes it more likely to be a lower lobe pneumonia. Look next at the hila which are normal. Look at the rest of the mediastinum. You will see a line on the right side of the neck running into the mediastinum. This is a right jugular line.

After you survey the lungs and mediastinum, look at the bones, soft tissues and area under the diaphragms. A survey of the bones will reveal fractures of both clavicles and lucencies within the mid shaft of the left humerus. The soft tissues are normal but there is some air trapped in the skin folds of the right axilla. There are no abnormalities beneath the diaphragm.

SUMMARY

The complications of myeloma shown on this film are pathological fractures, bone involvement, pneumonia and a pleural effusion, which could be secondary to infection or renal failure.

CXR 92

This 22-year-old woman presented with central chest pain relieved on leaning forwards. She had had a recent cough and cold, but was otherwise usually fit and well. What is the diagnosis?

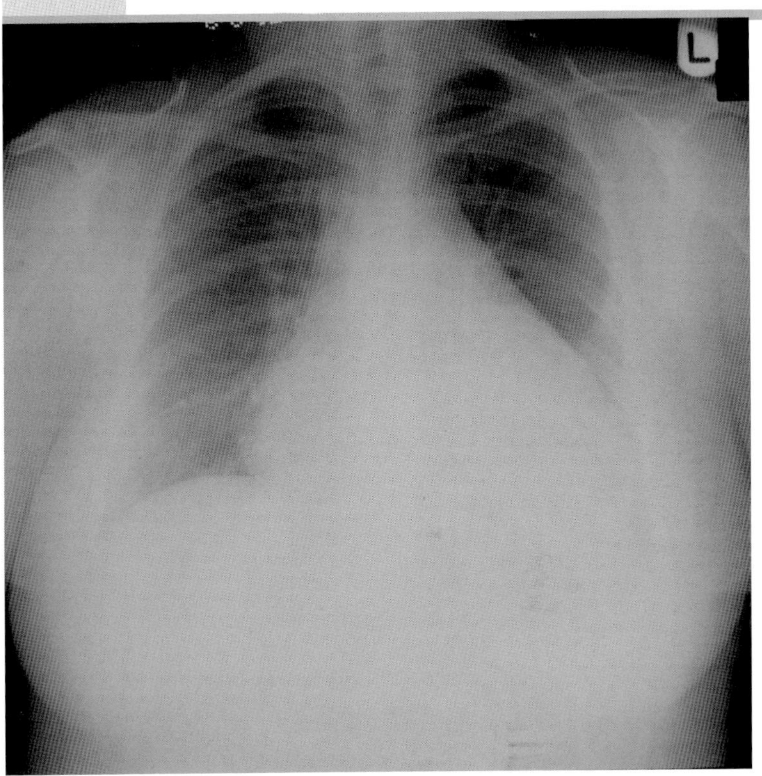

Initial impression

There is enlargement of the heart shadow.

Interpretation

The heart size appears increased. The left border of the heart is straightened and the heart looks triangular. The lung fields look normal.

When you notice an enlarged heart in a young person you need to examine the shape of the heart and also look at the lung fields for prominence of the blood vessels. In a young person, abnormalities of the heart shadow may indicate a congenital heart abnormality. An atrial septal defect would be expected to cause prominence of the blood vessels within the lung in view of the increased blood flow through these vessels. However, the lung fields in this case are normal. Other causes of an abnormal heart shadow can be related to the pericardium or abnormalities from other areas of the mediastinum extending downwards, such as enlarged lymph nodes or an enlarged thymus.

In a pericardial effusion, the fluid is surrounding the heart, so the heart appears globally enlarged and triangular, as in this film. A post-viral pericardial effusion is the most likely diagnosis here and this was confirmed at echocardiography.

SUMMARY

Pericardial effusion.

CXR 93

This is the film of a 67-year-old retired gardener, with known lung cancer. What complications have developed?

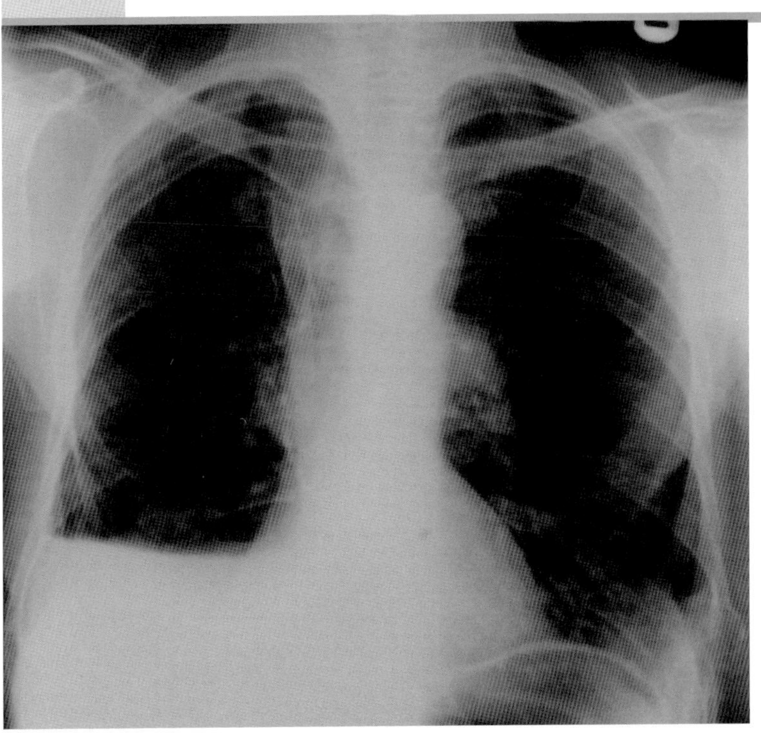

Initial impression

Straight white line at the right base. Mesh work along the mediastinum.

Interpretation

The right hemidiaphragm is obscured, and there is an area of whiteness with a straight upper border. This suggests a hydropneumothorax (air and fluid in the pleural space). The air can best be appreciated on the lateral edge, where there is an absence of lung markings, and the film appears slightly darker. Look at the ribs, the right 6th rib has been resected, an indication of previous thoracic surgery. There is metallic meshwork projected over the right side of the mediastinum, in the line of the superior vena cava.

Did you do a full survey of the ribs, and identify the other rib abnormality, at the left base? The 9th rib laterally has an area of expansion and destruction, in keeping with a bone metastasis.

This lady had surgery to remove a right-sided lung cancer, but she unfortunately has developed metastatic disease, and a local recurrence leading to superior vena caval obstruction. The hydropneumothorax is a result of recent drainage of her pleural effusion, performed for symptomatic relief.

SUMMARY

Hydropneumothorax, previous thoracotomy, superior vena caval stent and rib metastasis.

CXR 94

This 62-year-old stone cutter had this film taken as part of a private medical health check. He was subsequently referred to his local chest physician. What is the likely diagnosis?

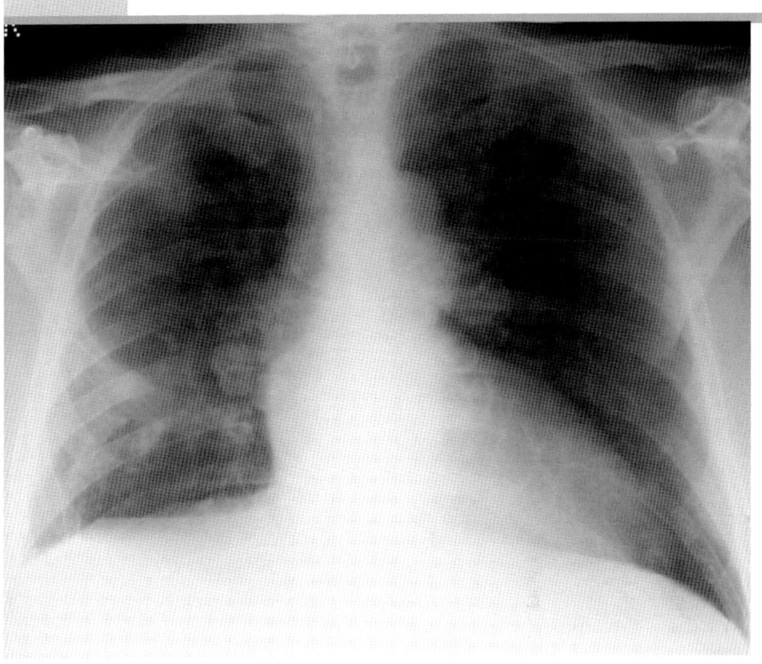

Initial impression

Abnormally shaped enlarged hilar areas.

Interpretation

There are oval densities, of around 1–3 cm in diameter, projected over the hilar regions on both sides of the mediastinum. These densities are not homogeneous, but have dense margins, which therefore must be calcified. This marginal calcification is termed egg shell calcification. This narrows the differential diagnosis. An important clue is given in the history, as he has been a stone cutter. Occupational exposure to stone dust can produce silicosis, which may cause lung changes and/or this form of hilar calcification. Other causes include sarcoidosis and treated lymphoma. Tuberculosis would tend to form solid calcified nodal masses, not the egg shell form.

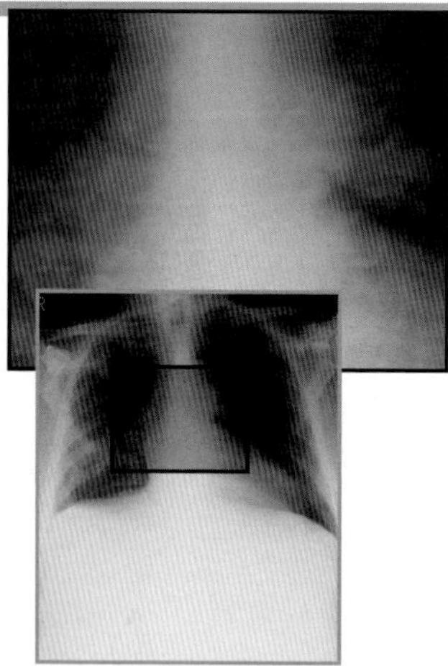

SUMMARY

Silicosis, an occupational lung disease.

CXR 95

This is the film of a 65-year-old smoker with a 1-month history of cough and breathlessness. What is the diagnosis?

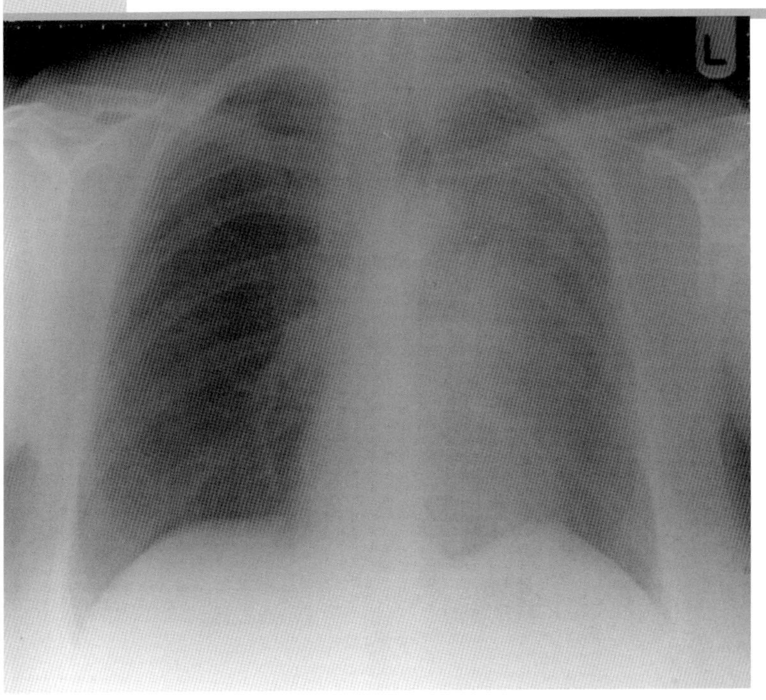

Initial impression

Abnormal white lung on the left and abnormal mediastinum.

Interpretation

There is increased opacity in the left chest, most dense in the upper portions and less marked in the lower zones. In addition, there are volume loss changes in the left chest, with shift of the trachea, and a rather angular type of elevation of the hemidiaphragm known as tenting (arrow). The mediastinum also appears abnormal, with loss of definition of the aortic arch. This volume loss and the distribution of the whiteness is typical of a left upper lobe collapse. The diaphragm remains clearly defined. The presence of collapse can be due to an endoluminal blockage – either a tumour or sometimes an inhaled foreign body. A bronchoscopy is indicated.

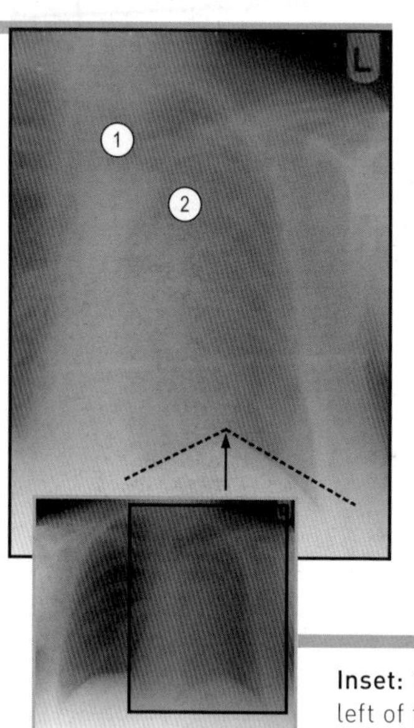

Inset: 1. Tracheal shift. 2. Loss of contours on the left of the mediastinum.

SUMMARY

Left upper lobe collapse.

CXR 96

This 59-year-old ex-coalminer had a film taken before an operation because of his breathlessness. What is the likely cause of the film appearance?

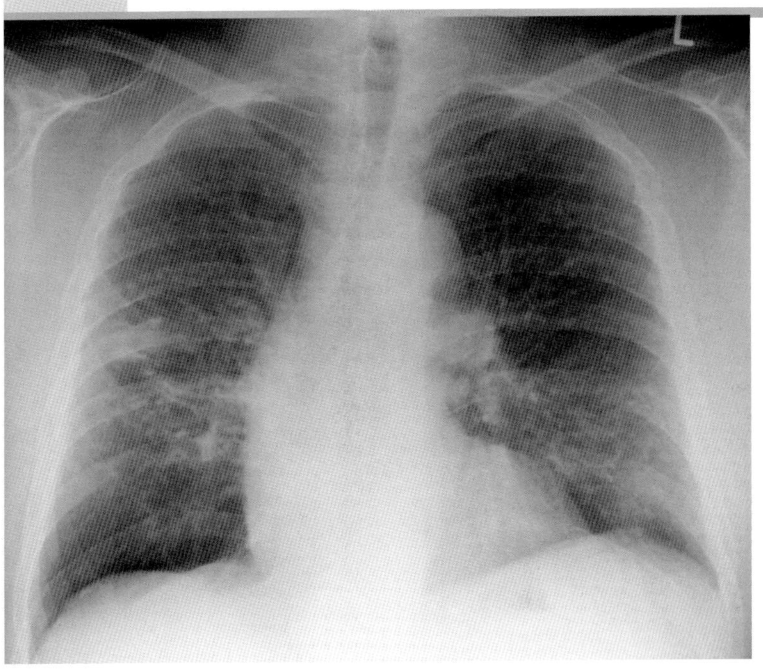

Initial impression

White lungs.

Interpretation

The lung fields are abnormally white. If you look closely at the lung fields you will see that this is due to the presence of numerous small vague circular shadows. Look closely at these shadows. Most of them are between 3–4 mm in diameter but in the right upper zone some of them have coalesced to form roughly circular shadows with a diameter of greater than 10 mm.

The patient has complicated coal worker's pneumoconiosis. The small circular lesions (less than 10 mm diameter) are typical of simple pneumoconiosis. The pneumoconiosis is defined as complicated if there are lesions of over 10 mm diameter present.

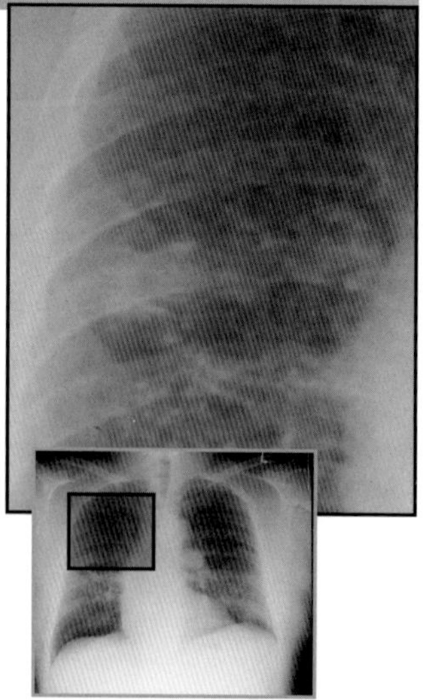

SUMMARY

Complicated coal worker's pneumoconiosis.

CXR 97

This 40-year-old man is in casualty following a serious road traffic accident. What features can you describe on the film?

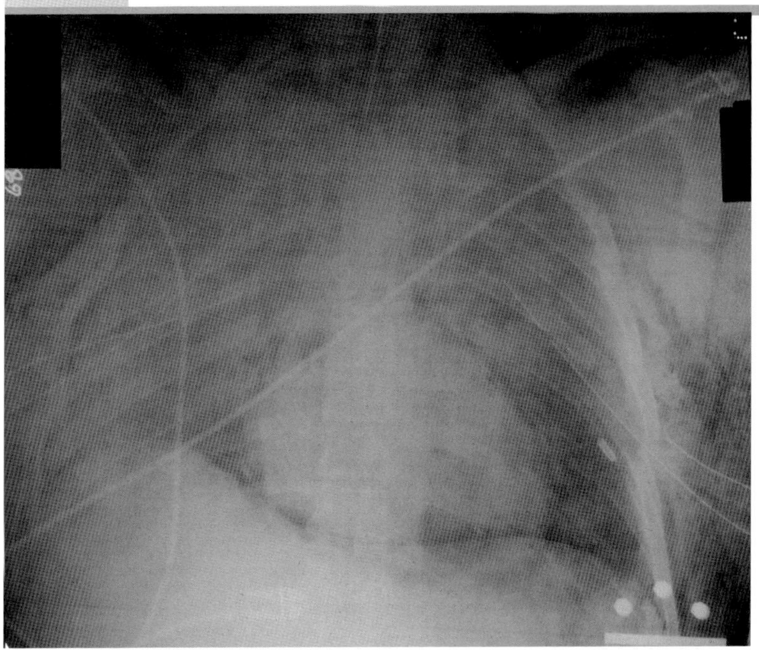

Initial impression

Extensive whiteness of both lungs.

Interpretation

This patient is obviously unwell. There is an endotracheal tube in situ and ECG leads are attached to the chest. Further inspection shows two chest drains on the right side with a further two chest drains on the left. You can also make out the dense tip of a tube in the left lower zone. This is a nasogastric tube, which has been misplaced.

You now have to consider the causes of a generalized white lung. Remember the history of trauma which would make pulmonary contusions highly likely, as a deceleration injury. Further causes are acute respiratory distress syndrome (ARDS), severe pulmonary oedema or aspiration pneumonia. The patchy whiteness in the lungs could be due to any of these causes.

Look at the rest of the film. You can see a streaky dark shadowing over the soft tissues of the chest wall and axillae. These dark shadows are lozenge shaped, an appearance typical of surgical emphysema (gas in the soft tissues). In this case it is a complication of the patient's traumatic pneumothorax, where air from the lung has escaped through the chest wall.

Look at the bones. In this case you will see a flail segment of the right chest wall (i.e. ribs with two fractures separating them completely from the chest wall). A subtle white line is also seen around the heart. This is a pneumopericardium.

SUMMARY

Intubated patient with bilateral chest drains, a misplaced nasogastric tube, surgical emphysema, flail chest and pnuemopericardium. Pulmonary contusions, pulmonary oedema or aspiration are all potential causes for the patchy shadowing within the lungs.

CXR 98

This 39-year-old man presented with asthma-like symptoms and fever. Full blood count showed a peripheral eosinophilia. What does the film show?

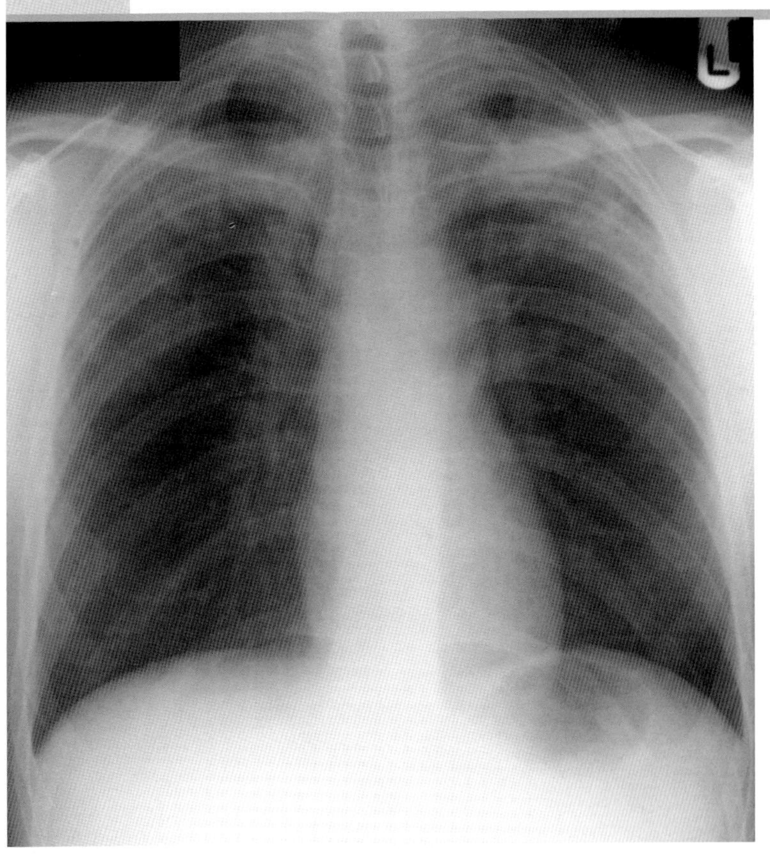

Initial impression

Bilateral whiteness in the lung apices.

Interpretation

This film demonstrates the importance of looking at the lung apices, since abnormalities are often obscured by the overlying ribs. In this case you can see increased shadowing. This is especially prominent on the left side, but close inspection also shows increased shadowing on the right.

With unilateral apical shadowing you should always think of tuberculosis. Bilateral apical shadowing is much less common and should make you consider systemic causes. In this case the diagnosis was eosinophilic pneumonia. You cannot make this diagnosis from the film alone. The important point is to remember to look at the apices in detail.

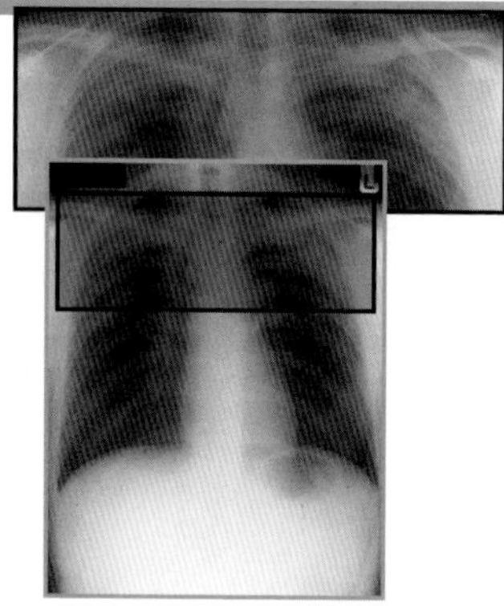

SUMMARY

Eosinophilic pneumonia.

CXR 99

This 53-year-old woman gave a 3-month history of increasing swelling of the ankles. On examination she had a raised jugular venous pressure. What is your interpretation of the film?

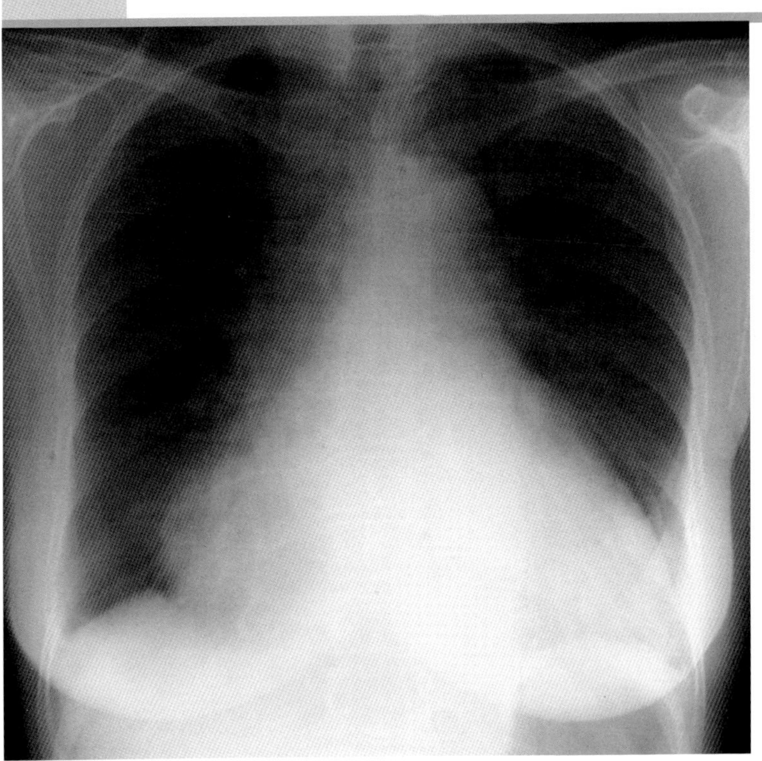

Initial impression

Abnormally shaped, enlarged heart.

Interpretation

The first thing to notice is that the heart is big since it is more than half the thoracic diameter. Once you have spotted this you need to decide which part of the heart is enlarged. As a general rule, enlargement of the heart on the left side of the vertebral column is due to enlargement of one or both ventricles, and enlargement to the right of the vertebral column, due to enlargement of either or both atria. In this case the left side has a more normal shape and the abnormal part of the heart lies on the right side of the vertebral column. This indicates a left or right atrial abnormality. The left atrium lies at the back, and would cause other changes, such as splaying of the carina to an angle of more than 90° and signs of pulmonary oedema. These features are not present – the carina and lung fields both look normal, so the enlargement is likely to be due to an enlarged right atrium. This woman had an enlarged right atrium because of tricuspid valve disease. This was confirmed by echocardiography. The ankle swelling was due to the right heart abnormality.

SUMMARY

Right atrial enlargement due to tricuspid valve disease.

CXR 100

This 58-year-old man who had never smoked complained of pleuritic chest pain of 2 days' duration. He also gave a history of haemoptysis. This film was taken in the emergency department. What does it show?

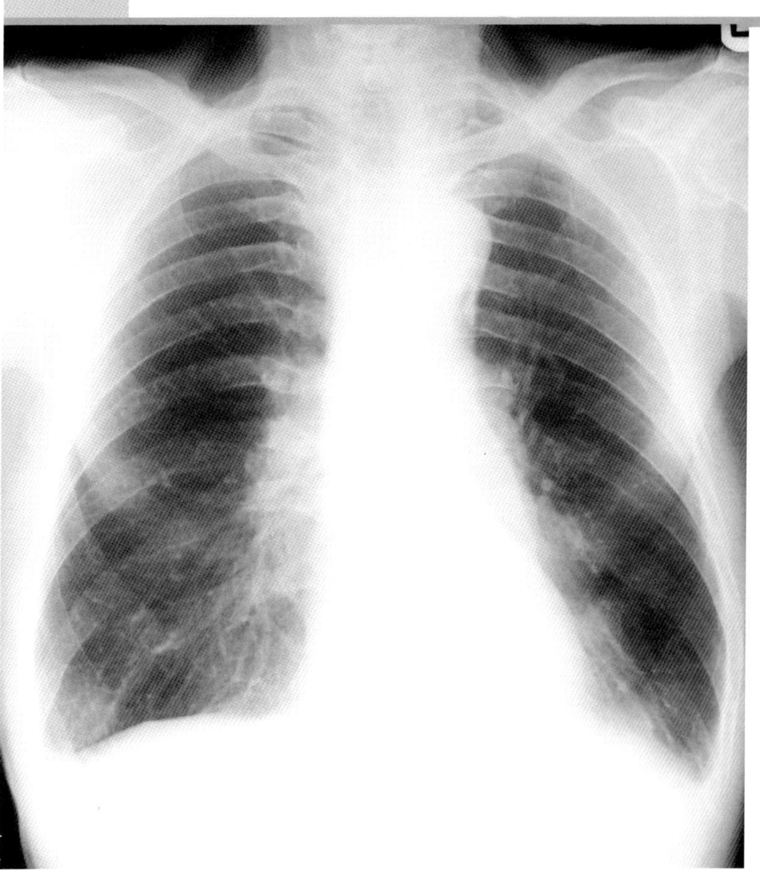

Initial impression

No obvious abnormality.

Interpretation

A quick look at this film shows no obvious abnormalities. You need to look at areas where abnormalities are easily missed. Look at the apices, which in this film are normal. Look at the diaphragms. Usually you are able to clearly see the left and right hemidiaphragm. In this film the left hemidiaphragm is not clearly visible, especially in the area behind the heart. This should alert you to the possibility of left lower lobe collapse, since the left lower lobe will collapse against the medial end of the left hemidiaphragm, blurring its border. To confirm the presence of left lower lobe collapse you need to look carefully at the area behind the heart. When the left lower lobe collapses it forms a dense triangular area behind the heart. This is the so-called sail sign and is just visible in this film.

If you follow the aortic knuckle downwards you will identify a tortuous descending aorta, a common feature and not a cause for concern in this age group. There is no diaphragmatic or mediastinal shift, but the left sided ribs are closer together than on the right, especially anteriorly. The left lung is also slightly darker than the right as the left upper lobe has overinflated to compensate for the lower lobe collapse. There is a small left pleural effusion.

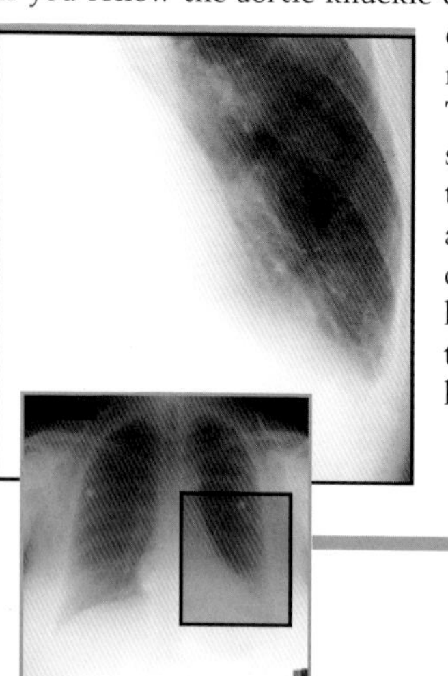

SUMMARY

Left lower lobe collapse. This can, as in this case, occur in the context of infection, but a bronchoscopy is advised to exclude endoluminal masses or foreign bodies.

Index